Fundamental Nursing Skills

This book is dedicated to my late mother Noreen,
my inspiration, motivation, confidante and best friend.
A very brave and compassionate lady to the end.

fundamental
nursing skills

Edited by **Penelope Ann Hilton** SEN, SRN, RMN,
DIPN (LOND), FETC, BSc (HONS), MMEDSCI, RNT

Lecturer in Nursing, University of Sheffield

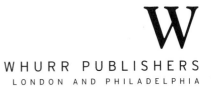

WHURR PUBLISHERS
LONDON AND PHILADELPHIA

© 2004 Whurr Publishers Ltd
First published 2004
by Whurr Publishers Ltd
19b Compton Terrace
London N1 2UN England and
325 Chestnut Street, Philadelphia PA 19106 USA

Reprinted 2004

British Library Cataloguing in Publication Data

A catalogue record for this book
is available from the British Library.

ISBN 1 86156 416 3

Typeset by Adrian McLaughlin, a@microguides.net
Printed and bound in the UK by Athenæum Press Limited, Gateshead, Tyne & Wear

Contents

Acknowledgements

First of all my eternal gratitude must be expressed to Rose for her unending perseverance and support. I would like to thank the many enlightened health care practitioners and students from the Royal Hallamshire Hospital, Sheffield, the Northern General Hospital, Sheffield and Chesterfield & North Derbyshire Royal Hospital, who contributed to the original research to verify the need for and content of such a text way back in 1994, and for their continued enthusiasm and input. I would also like to thank the many clients and relatives who shared their critical opinions; my colleagues whom I somehow managed to press-gang into authorship; the student nurses who very kindly passed judgement on the emerging chapters, not least Kerry Atkin, Emma Cornell, Fiona Maris; Sophie Kerslake for the brilliant illustrations; and Joanne Chilvers, Joint Course Leader for the Advanced Diploma in Nursing Studies programme at the University of Sheffield, for her critical reading of the final manuscript.

Preface

This book has arisen primarily in response to the increasing concern expressed about the perceived lack of ability in both students and newly qualified staff nurses to perform clinical skills. This deficit has been largely attributed to the advent of Project 2000 and the subsequent move of nurse education into Higher Education. Innovations in nursing such as the Nursing Process, Nursing Models and new methods of organizing care delivery, each with their emphasis on providing individualized nursing care, may also have exacerbated this problem. These initiatives have largely resulted in the demise of procedure manuals as a source of reference in many clinical areas. Consequently nurses and the increasing number of health care workers in new roles such as cadet nurses, health care assistants and generic ward practitioners no longer have an easily accessible source of reference in the clinical arena. This is particularly problematic when they are faced with undertaking a procedure for the first time.

The intention of this book is to redress this deficit by:

1 outlining the elements of essential nursing procedures in a readily accessible format
2 providing the rationale for the recommended actions
3 promoting evidence-based practice.

This book is unique in that it encourages the reader to keep a record of achievement in relation to clinical skill competence. It also differs from existing publications in that it is presented in a more readily accessible and user-friendly format for the busy clinician. Further, this text may be of benefit to lay persons undertaking the main carer role in the home setting.

The selection of skills for inclusion is based on extensive consultation with experienced clinicians, students, clients and their significant others as well as teachers of nursing. Each procedure has been carefully researched to provide a contemporary foundation for practice. The book is the first of a series which aims to promote professional and personal development from novice through to expert in sequential stages. References and further reading are offered at the conclusion of each chapter.

The inherent danger in producing books of this nature is that they may be perceived to be encouraging a task-orientated approach to patient care. In acknowledging this potential the chapters have been structured around the Activities of Living (Roper et al 2000) to encourage the reader to view each of the skills as an intricate part of holistic individualized care. The book also contains a rapid reference section of common terminology, conversion tables, laboratory results and other, equally useful, information.

Whilst every attempt has been made throughout the text to reflect contemporary practices, the reader is reminded that practice will continue to develop in the light of new evidence and changing policy. A commitment to lifelong learning is therefore essential.

Penelope Ann Hilton
December 2003

Reference

Roper N, Logan WW, Tierney A (2000) The Roper-Logan-Tierney Model of Nursing: The Activities of Living Model. Edinburgh: Churchill Livingstone.

Contributors

Samantha Athorn RGN, STH Movement and Handling Key Trainer, Practice and Professional Development Sister, Royal Hallamshire Hospital, Sheffield

Julie Foster RN (Adult), DipN (Sheffield Hallam), Senior Staff Nurse, Gynaecological Directorate, Royal Hallamshire Hospital, Sheffield

Penelope Ann Hilton SEN, SRN, RMN, DipN (Lond), FETC, BSc (Hons), MMedSci, RNT Lecturer in Nursing, University of Sheffield

Alyson Hoyles RGN, SCM, DipN (Lond), PGCEA, RNT, BEd (Hons), MSc (Nursing) Nursing Lecturer, University of Sheffield

Sheila Lees RGN, MMedSci, BA (Hons), RCNT, DipN (Lond), FETC Nursing Lecturer, University of Sheffield

Beverly Levy MA, BSc (Hons), RGN, RCNT, Cert Ed (FE), RNT Nursing Lecturer, University of Sheffield

Carol Pollard ONC, RGN, DipN (Lond), Cert Ed (FE), BA (Hons), MMedSci, RNT Nursing Lecturer, University of Sheffield

Neal Seymour MA (Ed), BA (Hons), RSCN, RGN, RNT Lecturer/Practitioner, Sheffield Children's Hospital/University of Sheffield

Helen Taylor RGN, RMN, RNMH, BSc (Hons), MMedSci, RNT Nursing Lecturer, University of Sheffield

Catherine Waskett RGN, BSc (Hons), MSc, ONC, Lecturer in Nursing, University of Sheffield

Introduction

In 1859 Florence Nightingale suggested that 'The elements of nursing are all but unknown'. It could be argued that this statement remains true today: some groups maintain that nursing is about keeping clients clean and well nourished; others that it is about making clients feel safe; others focus purely on the psychological needs of clients; and yet others think that it is about carrying out physical tasks delegated by, but remaining under the auspices of, doctors (Hilton 1997).

In looking back down the well-trodden path it can be seen that over the past 150 years or so nursing has slowly evolved from something that was considered essentially women's work, which could be undertaken by any 'good woman', was largely concerned with caring for the sick, and with providing the best environment for nature to take its course, to being something that is very complex, skilled and sometimes highly technical, involving health education and promotion as well as meeting a wide variety of illness-related needs of clients. It is now an occupation that attracts both men and women whose pay constitutes more than a bottle of gin (Hilton 1997).

Indeed, many now contend that nursing has reached the epitome, that long-strived-for goal of professional recognition (Clay 1987), as it now has an academic, secular training programme, a Code of Professional Conduct (see Appendix I) and its own regulating body, the Nurses and Midwives Council. It is a profession that is clearly distinct from medicine, where registered nurses are considered autonomous, accountable practitioners who work from a soundly researched knowledge base and whose practice is for the benefit of others.

The majority of changes that have occurred in nursing and other emergent professions allied to medicine, such as physiotherapy and occupational therapy, have occurred as a result of changing health care needs, technological advances and a plethora of new knowledge as well as changes in societal attitudes, values and beliefs and an increasing cultural milieu. We now live in times of continuing change and advancement.

Consequently health care, and therefore nursing, cannot remain a static entity. It must move, develop and evolve in the light of societal changes along with its other related disciplines.

In order to enable effective response, to provide direction to influence health care policy and legislation, to assist in determining further workforce needs, and to inform resource management the Royal College of Nursing (RCN) has recently undertaken a scoping exercise. It defined nursing as 'the use of clinical judgement and the provision of care to enable people to promote, improve, maintain or recover health or, when death is inevitable, to die peacefully' (RCN 2003:1). This has come at a time when the current government is seeking to contain costs, destabilize the professions and merge professional boundaries with the ultimate aim of promoting better interprofessional working and, thus, higher standards and more cost-effective but better-quality health care.

As such, a much greater emphasis is being placed on the promotion and maintenance of health and well-being. However, a word of caution: this definition advanced by the RCN, and the assumptions on which it is based, should not be viewed in isolation. As with many of the previous definitions of nursing offered and indeed the sometimes radical changes in nursing and health care that have taken place in recent years, to date there has been no client involvement in its conception or development.

However, despite presenting a little background to nursing and health care today, it is not the purpose of this text to dwell on definitions of health and illness or to debate the politics of health care, but to provide practical direction in day-to-day clinical experiences. It would therefore seem prudent to reflect on current practice, part of which is about assessing client care needs.

Assessment and the nursing process

In order to determine a client's care needs, assessment is a crucial first step. If a client's normal routines, patterns and behaviours are not explored and compared with their current health care status and abilities, significant aspects of care need may be omitted or care may be provided that the client does not require. In doing so, there is a risk of jeopardizing their independence and losing their trust and confidence. Assessment is the first stage of a four-stage cyclical process generally referred to as the 'Nursing Process' (Yura and Walsh 1967), a concept developed in the USA during the early 1980s. The other three stages are planning, implementing, and evaluation, though other writers include data collection and diagnosis as separate stages.

Whilst the emphasis appears to be on nursing, it can be argued that it is equally applicable to any profession claiming to provide a service and encountering a client for the first time. For those interested in exploring the historical development of this concept further, some key texts can be found at the end of this section.

Assessment includes collecting all relevant information and then determining the client's actual or potential problems. From this information care can then be planned in full consultation with the client, their significant others and other members of the multidisciplinary team as appropriate. Care planning should be clearly documented and include the goals of care – that is, what it is we are striving to achieve – making sure, of course, that these are both realistic and achievable, along with precise details of how they are going to be achieved.

For example, Fred has been admitted to an acute medical setting with a very bad chest infection. On assessing his ability to breathe it is evident that he is experiencing difficulty expectorating his sputum; that is, he is unable to cough up the secretions from his lungs that are resulting from his infection. The goal of care may be that Fred will expectorate freely prior to discharge. The care then might include:

- ensuring that Fred drinks a minimum of two litres of fluid per day
- ensuring that he has a ready supply of sputum pots and tissues
- referring him to the physiotherapist
- providing chest percussion a least three times a day
- instructing him in how to undertake deep breathing exercises to promote expectoration
- ensuring that he undertakes these a minimum of three times a day prior to meals
- providing mouthwashes every four hours and on request.

Everyone involved in Fred's care is therefore very clear about his care needs and can then go on to implement these without constantly having to check with Fred, the physiotherapist or other colleagues – provided of course that the instructions are clear and comprehensible (see the section on 'Record keeping' in Chapter 6).

It is also useful to include measurements wherever possible as this can help us to evaluate whether or not Fred has achieved the desired goals of care later.

The nursing process and nursing models

Whilst the nursing process offers a systematic way of looking at care delivery, on its own it is not particularly useful as it does not give any indication as to what to assess. It indicates that care should be planned, implemented and evaluated but again offers little direction as to how to do this. Consequently a number of practitioners and nurse theorists have offered theoretical frameworks or models. One such model is the 'Activities of Living Model', proposed by Nancy Roper, Winifred Logan and Alison Tierney (1996). Basing their ideas on previous work by Maslow (1958) and Virginia Henderson (1960), and Nancy Roper herself, Roper, Logan and Tierney set out to describe what they believed everyday living involves for individuals, and from this identify the necessary components of nursing.

In very simple terms their model can be summarized as consisting of four components, which all contribute to individuality in living, namely (1) the lifespan continuum from conception to death; (2) 12 activities of living (listed below); (3) five factors that influence each of these activities, that is physical, psychological, sociocultural, environmental and politicoeconomic; and (4) a dependence/independence continuum.

The 12 activities of living are:

1 breathing
2 mobilizing
3 personal cleansing and dressing
4 maintaining a safe environment
5 eating and drinking
6 communicating
7 dying
8 eliminating
9 maintaining body temperature
10 expressing sexuality
11 working and playing
12 sleeping.

According to Roper and her co-workers (2000), by assessing each of these aspects it is possible to determine a person's individual nursing and health care needs and in doing so determine priorities of care. For example, when assessing an adult with an enduring mental health problem such as chronic depression, eating and drinking may be the priority of care, whereas if caring for a very young child, maintaining a safe environment might be the most urgent concern.

To return for a moment to Fred, clearly the illustration presented is of just one aspect of his care needs related to the physical side of the 'activity of breathing'. In order to deliver holistic care (i.e. making sure that all his care needs are met), each factor of each activity must be assessed and his level of independence or dependence determined. So, for example, Fred may also be very anxious about not being able to expectorate his sputum and may think that if he cannot cough it out he will die. This illustrates how the activities, in reality, often overlap. By providing this simple framework, however, Roper, Logan and Tierney help to direct our thinking in a more logical, sequential way and if every aspect of each activity is covered when clients are assessed a clear picture of their individual needs should emerge without the omission of any important points.

Whilst some might argue that Roper, Logan and Tierney's model is not appropriate in caring for clients with learning difficulties or mental health problems, it is in fact the most widely used framework in Europe regardless of setting. If utilized to its fullest extent, it can usefully direct learners in any field of health care. Therefore, the remainder of this text is structured around their 12 activities of living to help readers to relate the theory to everyday practice.

Each of the following 12 chapters offers: an introduction to the activity; common terminology related to that activity; points to consider when assessing the activity; followed by fundamental care skills related to that activity. Appendix I is a rapid reference section, which gives a detailed glossary to support the main text, normal values and other such useful information. Appendix II provides an opportunity for readers to record their achievements.

Finally, as a point of note, whilst acknowledging the variety of terms in use, as well as possible gender issues, for ease and continuity the term 'client' has been used throughout this text.

References and further reading

Aggleton P, Chalmers H (2000) Nursing Models and Nursing Practice, 2nd edn. Basingstoke: Macmillan Press.

Christenson P, Kenny J (1995) Nursing Process: Application of Conceptual Models. St Louis, MI: CV Mosby.

Clay T (1987) Nurses, Power and Politics. London: Heinemann.

Hawthorne DL, Yurkovich NJ (1995) Science, technology, caring and the professions: are they compatible? Journal of Advanced Nursing 21(6): 1087–1091.

Henderson V (1960) Basic Principles of Nursing Care. London: ICN.

Hilton PA (1997) Theoretical perspectives of nursing: a review of the literature. Journal of Advanced Nursing 26: 1211–1220.

Marriner A (1979) The Nursing Process. St Louis, MI: CV Mosby.

Maslow A (1958) Hierarchy of Needs, cited in Maslow A (1968) Towards a Psychology of Being. New York: Rheinhold.

Murphy K, Cooney A, Casey D, Connor M, O'Connor J, Dineen B (2000) The Roper, Logan and Tierney (1996) model: perceptions and operationalisation of the model in psychiatric nursing within a Health Board in Ireland. Journal of Advanced Nursing 31(6): 1333–1341.

Nightingale F (1859) Notes on Nursing: What it is and what it is not. London: Duckworth (reprinted 1952).

Nurses and Midwives Council (2002) Code of Professional Conduct. London: NMC.

Roper N, Logan WW, Tierney A (1996) The Elements of Nursing, 4th edn. Edinburgh: Churchill Livingstone.

Roper N, Logan WW, Tierney A (2000) The Roper-Logan-Tierney Model of Nursing: The Activities of Living Model. Edinburgh: Churchill Livingstone.

Royal College of Nursing (2003) Defining Nursing. London: RCN.

Thomas B, Hardy S (eds) (1997) Stuart and Sundeen's Mental Health Nursing – Principles and Practice. St Louis, MI: CV Mosby.

Wimpenny P (2002) The meaning of models of nursing to practising nurses. Journal of Advanced Nursing 40(3): 346–354.

Yura H, Walsh M (1967) The Nursing Process. Norwalk, Connecticut: Appleton-Century-Crofts.

Chapter 1

Breathing

Penelope Ann Hilton

Introduction

The process of external respiration (breathing) consists of two stages, namely *inspiration*, inhaling (breathing in) air in order to extract the oxygen from the air, and *expiration*, exhaling (breathing out) in order to expel carbon dioxide. Oxygen is required by the body to release energy at cell level so that the individual can participate in activities. The release of such energy through metabolism produces carbon dioxide as a waste product that must be expelled from the body. The presence of carbon dioxide in the blood plays a key role in maintaining respiratory function and in maintaining homeostasis by regulating the pH of the blood (acid–base balance). A pH value between 7.35 and 7.45 is essential for normal body functioning.

Breathing is essential to life. The ability to undertake a swift assessment of the client's ability to breathe and instigate removal of an obstruction and/or rescue breathing if needed is therefore crucial (see 'Maintenance of an airway' and 'Artificial respiration'). A full assessment of the person's ability to breathe should be undertaken once adequate respiratory function has been restored.

There are several important structural differences between adults and children that influence respiration, including the shape of the chest at birth, shape and angle of the ribs and elastic properties of the lung tissue. The nasal passages and trachea of infants and young children are narrower and can therefore be more easily obstructed. They also have less alveolar surface area for gaseous exchange. These latter points are extremely important when attempting to remove an obstruction or provide effective rescue breathing. It is, therefore, crucial to be familiar with the different techniques for these client groups.

Factors that may affect breathing may be:

- *physical*, arising from alteration in the structure, function or processes of the respiratory and associated systems
- *psychological*, such as anxiety and stress
- *sociocultural*, for example smoking

- *environmental*, including pollution and allergies
- *politico-economic*, for example lack of finances for heating.

The remainder of this chapter gives the common terminology associated with the activity of breathing, points to consider when assessing an individual's breathing, how to monitor respiratory rate and peak flow, airway maintenance, monitoring of expectorant, obtaining specimens and disposing of sputum, administration of oxygen, and rescue breathing. The chapter concludes with references and further reading.

Common terminology

Aerobic	With oxygen
Anaerobic	Without oxygen
Anoxia	No oxygen reaching the brain
Apnoea	Absence of breathing
Apnoeustic breathing	Prolonged gasping inspiration and short inefficient expiration
Asthmatic breathing	Difficulty on expiration with an audible expiratory wheeze. Caused by spasm of the respiratory passages and partial blockage by increased mucus secretion
Biot's respirations	Periods of hyperpnoea occurring in normal respiration. Sometimes seen in clients with meningitis
Bradypnoea	Slow but regular breathing. Normal in sleep but may be a sign of opiate use, alcohol indulgence or brain tumour
Cheyne-Stokes respirations	Gradual cycle of increased rate and depth followed by gradual decrease with the pattern repeating every 45 seconds to three minutes. Also associated with periods of apnoea, particularly in the dying
Cyanosis	A bluish appearance of the skin and mucous membranes caused by inadequate oxygenation
Dyspnoea	Difficulty breathing
Expiration	The act of breathing out
Haemoptysis	Blood in the sputum
Homeostasis	The automatic self-regulation of man to maintain the normal state of the body under a variety of environmental conditions
Hypercapnia	High partial pressure of carbon dioxide
Hyperpnoea	Deep breathing with marked use of abdominal muscles
Hyperventilation	Increased rate and depth of breathing
Hypoventilation	Irregular, slow, shallow breathing

Hypoxia	A lack of oxygen concentration
Hypoxaemia	A lack of oxygen in the blood
Inspiration	The act of breathing in
Kussmaul's respirations	Increased respiratory rate (above 20 rpm), increased depth, panting laboured breathing. Causes include diabetic ketoacidosis and renal failure
Orthopnoea	The ability to breath easily only when in an upright position
Perfusion	The flow of oxygenated blood to the tissues
Stridor	A harsh, vibrating, shrill sound produced during respiration. Usually indicates an obstruction
Tachypnoea	Increased rate of breathing
Tracheostomy	Making of an opening into the trachea or windpipe
Ventilation	The movement of air in and out of the lungs

Assessing an individual's ability to breathe

Remember that assessment of breathing is only part of a holistic nursing assessment and should not be undertaken in isolation without reference to or consideration of the client's other activities of living.

The specific points to be considered when assessing an individual's breathing include:

- *Physical*
  Respiratory rate
    depth
    sounds
    pattern/rhythm
  Presence of cough
    productive
    unproductive
  Sputum
    colour
    consistency
    amount
    smell
  Degree of effort, use of accessory muscles (e.g. shoulders/neck)
  Nasal flaring, which is usually a sign of increased effort, particularly in infants
  Sternal recession, the sinking in of sternum during inspiration, particularly in infants
  Tracheal tug, the sinking in of the soft tissues above the sternum and between the clavicles during inspiration, particularly in infants
  Intercostal recession, the sinking in of the soft tissues between the ribs during inspiration

Facial expressions

Colour of skin/mucous membranes – mottling, pallor, cyanosis

Presence of scars

Shape of thorax, symmetry of movement

Evidence of external/internal injury

Position adopted by client and influence of body position on breathing

Pain related to inspiration/expiration/movement

Breathes through mouth and/or nose

Clubbing of finger ends

Head bobbing, that is, forward movement of head on inspiration in a
   sleeping or exhausted infant is a sign of breathing difficulty

Status of hypoxic drive, that is, is the client retaining carbon dioxide?

- *Psychological*
  Stress
  Anxiety
  Depression
  Hysteria
  Irritability
  Confusion

- *Sociocultural*
  Level of support from family/external agencies
  Smoking
  Health beliefs/values
  Hobbies/pastimes
  Level of family support

- *Environmental*
  Pollution, such as dust mites and pollen
  Cold, damp or foggy weather
  Type of accommodation
  Stairs to climb
  Work related

- *Politico-economic*
  Limited finances
  Employed/unemployed
  Poor heating
  Poor diet

- *Past history*
  Past illnesses related/unrelated
  Recent holiday abroad
  Family difficulties
  Powers of recovery
  Knowledge of condition

Monitoring respiratory rate

Monitoring a client's respiration rate is essential to facilitate the evaluation of medical treatment and nursing interventions.

Equipment

A digital watch or watch with a second hand, together with an appropriate chart for recording, is required. The procedures and rationales are given below.

Procedure	Rationale
Explain procedure and ensure adequate understanding	Promote client co-operation and obtain informed consent, though this step is often omitted where there is a danger that the person may voluntarily control their breathing and thus alter the rate
Count respirations as chest rises and falls for a period of one minute	To monitor rate and compare to norm values New-born: 30-80 rpm Early childhood: 20-40 rpm Late childhood: 15-25 rpm Adult male: 14-18 rpm Adult female: 16-20 rpm Pulse-to-respiration ratio = 5:1
Observe depth of respirations	To monitor depth and compare to norm – usually shallow and effortless
Listen for breath sounds, e.g. stridor, wheeze, rub, rattle	To monitor sounds and compare to norm – usually almost inaudible
Observe pattern of breathing and use of accessory muscles	To monitor pattern and compare to norm – usually effortless
Observe colour of skin/mucous membranes, e.g. pallor, cyanosis	To ensure that adequate oxygen is getting to the tissues (i.e. tissue perfusion)
Record rate on appropriate chart and report any abnormalities	Legal requirement to maintain documentation and safeguard client through good communications

Monitoring peak flow

Monitoring a client's peak flow levels gives an indication of respiratory function and facilitates objective evaluation of treatment, for example nebulizer therapy. A peak flow recording is defined as a measurement of the amount of air that can be forcibly exhaled and is used to monitor respiratory function. Bear in mind that peak flow measurement should *not* be attempted on patients in severe respiratory distress.

Equipment

The equipment needed to monitor peak flow consists of a peak flow meter and mouthpiece and an appropriate chart for recording the results. The procedures and rationales are given below.

Procedure	Rationale
Explain procedure and ensure adequate understanding	To promote client co-operation and obtain informed consent
Assist client into an upright position	To promote lung expansion
Fix mouthpiece to peak flow meter	To ensure correct assembly of equipment
Ensure the pointer is at zero	To ensure accurate reading is obtained
Hold meter, ensuring that fingers are clear of the scale and the holes in the base of the meter	To ensure accurate reading is obtained
Instruct client to take a deep breath	To fill lung fields to capacity with air to be exhaled
Instruct the client to hold the meter horizontally	To obtain accurate reading
Instruct client to place the mouthpiece in their mouth and close lips securely around it	To create a seal around the mouthpiece and thus prevent air leakage
Instruct client to exhale as hard as possible into the meter and sustain this for as long as possible	To expel as much air as possible
Note the number on the scale	To monitor peak flow and compare to the norm. Norm values depend on age, height and gender, e.g. Boy aged 9, 1.47 m = 350 litres/min 　　　Woman aged 30, 1.60 m = 475 litres/min 　　　Man aged 50, 1.75 m = 600 litres/min
Return pointer to zero	To prepare for second attempt
Repeat procedure twice more	To obtain highest score from three attempts
Reposition the client	To promote client comfort
Record scores on appropriate chart and report any deviation from the norm	Legal requirement to maintain documentation and safeguard the client through good communications
Wash mouthpiece in warm water with a mild detergent and dry thoroughly unless disposable	To prevent cross-infection

Maintenance of an airway

Airways must remain free from obstruction to enable effective respiratory function and thus sustain life. Remember, if the client has stopped breathing instigate artificial respirations immediately (see the section on 'Artificial respiration'). The procedures and rationales are given below.

Procedure	Rationale
Listen for breath sounds	Noisy laboured breathing or a stridor would indicate an obstruction
Observe chest and abdominal movement	Reverse movement of these, i.e. chest sucked in and abdomen protruding indicates an obstruction
Observe colour of skin/mucous membranes	Evidence of a blue tinge (cyanosis) is suggestive of an obstruction
ADULT (over 16 years) If you suspect an obstruction check in the client's mouth for any obvious obstruction, e.g. vomit, foreign body, etc. and remove same by sweeping the mouth with a finger. Great care should be taken not to push any foreign body further into the air passage. See also Chapter 5	Removal of an obvious obstruction will open the airways
CHILD (1–16 years)/**INFANT** (0–12 months) If the client is a child or infant only remove the obstruction if it is possible to do so *without* sweeping the mouth with a finger	Sweeping the mouth with a finger may cause serious trauma and/or further obstruct the airway
ADULT If unconscious tilt the head well back and lift the chin (see Figure 1.2a)	When unconscious the tongue may sag in the throat and block the airway. By tilting the head and lifting the chin the tongue will be lifted clear of the back of the throat. If airway clearance is not obtained try a jaw thrust (see Figure 1.2a)
CHILD If the child is unconscious gently lift the chin and tilt the head only slightly (i.e. sniffing position, see Figure 1.2b)	If the head of a child or infant is tilted too far back it will act to decrease the area of functional airway rather than maximize it. If airway clearance is not obtained try a jaw thrust (see Figure 1.2b)
INFANT The desirable degree of tilt in the infant is neutral (i.e. not tilted back, Figure 1.3)	

Procedure	Rationale
ADULT Place client in recovery position (see the section 'Moving and positioning clients' in Chapter 2) once normal respiratory function is restored	To maintain patient safety
CHILD/INFANT Assist the child to find a comfortable position once normal respiratory function is restored	A child/infant will often find the best position to maintain their airway and should not be forced into a position which is uncomfortable

Figure 1.1 (a) Head tilt and chin lift (adult); (b) Head tilt and chin lift (child)

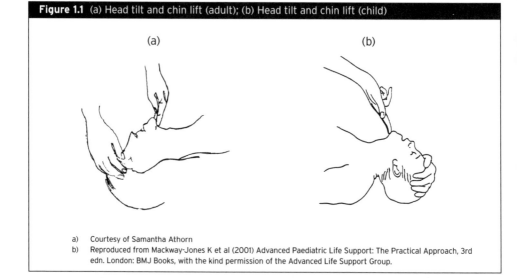

(a) (b)

a) Courtesy of Samantha Athorn
b) Reproduced from Mackway-Jones K et al (2001) Advanced Paediatric Life Support: The Practical Approach, 3rd edn. London: BMJ Books, with the kind permission of the Advanced Life Support Group.

Figure 1.2 (a) Jaw thrust (adult); (b) Jaw thrust (child)

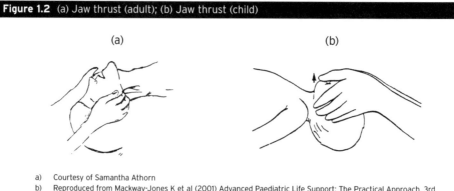

(a) (b)

a) Courtesy of Samantha Athorn
b) Reproduced from Mackway-Jones K et al (2001) Advanced Paediatric Life Support: The Practical Approach, 3rd edn. London: BMJ Books, with the kind permission of the Advanced Life Support Group.

Figure 1.3 Neutral (infant)

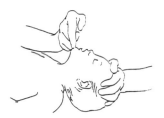

Reproduced from Mackway-Jones K et al (2001) Advanced Paediatric Life Support: The Practical Approach, 3rd edn. London: BMJ Books, with the kind permission of the Advanced Life Support Group.

Monitoring expectorant

Monitoring expectorations facilitates thorough assessment and evaluation of the client's condition and response to treatment. Expectorant refers to any secretions coughed out of the lungs and should not be confused with saliva (secretions from the mouth).

Equipment

The equipment required for monitoring consists of sputum pot, weighing scales (if available), appropriate chart for documenting results, and gloves. The procedures and rationales are given below.

Procedure	Rationale
Glove hands	To protect against infection
Observe colour	To monitor colour and compare to the norm. Yellow to green sputum indicates degree of infection. Putty or grey colour may indicate TB. Blood-streaked sputum may be caused by trauma or lung disease. Haemoptysis (blood in the sputum) is indicative of lung disease. Pink frothy sputum is indicative of heart disease/ pulmonary oedema.
Observe consistency	To monitor consistency and compare to the norm

Procedure	Rationale
Observe amount by weighing the sputum pot with the expectorant and subtracting the weight of an empty pot. If scales not available record amount as full pot, half pot, etc.	To measure the amount and compare to the norm. Weighing the expectorant gives an objective measure of the amount and is therefore more accurate and facilitates evaluation
Note any odour from the expectorant without directly inhaling over the pot	Directly inhaling over the pot may lead to inhalation of airborne micro-organisms
Record findings on appropriate chart and report any deviation from the norm	Legal requirement to maintain documentation and safeguard client safety through good communications
Dispose of sputum pot as directed in next section below	To prevent cross-infection
Provide client with a clean sputum pot indicating client's name and ensure an adequate supply of tissues	To maintain client comfort and facilitate evaluation
Advise client on the need to maintain hydration and oral hygiene (see Chapter 3) and offer assistance as necessary	To promote client comfort and reduce the risk of complications

Disposal of sputum/oral secretions

Safe disposal of sputum/oral secretions is essential to prevent spread of infection.

Equipment

The equipment required consists of sputum pot, waste bag for clinical waste, and gloves. The procedures and rationales are given below.

Procedure	Rationale
Monitor expectorant, as above, ensuring that any measurements and observations are recorded and reported prior to disposal	To ensure that the client's condition is monitored and to facilitate evaluation of condition
Replace lid on sputum pot and ensure tightly sealed	To prevent leakage of contents
Place in clinical waste bag and seal	To prevent leakage should lid become dislodged
Place in clinical waste bin for incineration	To prevent cross-infection
Wash and dry hands thoroughly	To prevent cross-infection
Provide client with a clean sputum pot indicating client's name and date	To maintain client comfort and facilitate evaluation

Obtaining a sputum specimen

An analysis of a sputum specimen will identify any abnormalities and provide direction for appropriate treatment.

Equipment

The equipment required consists of specimen pot with lid, clearly labelled with client details; request form signed by a doctor, and labelled with client details; specimen bag; tissues; and mouthwash/oral hygiene equipment. The procedures and rationales are given below.

Procedure	Rationale
Explain procedure to client	To increase client co-operation and obtain informed consent
Encourage and assist the client to cough into the specimen pot	Coughing expels the sputum from the lung fields
If experiencing difficulty in obtaining the specimen, gently percuss the client's back in collaboration with the physiotherapist	Gentle percussion dislodges sputum, making it easier to expel
Check that expectorant contains sputum	Test will be invalid if saliva is sent in error
Obtain assistance from physiotherapist if you encounter difficulties in obtaining specimen	Physiotherapists are trained specifically in techniques that may help to obtain a specimen
Replace lid on pot ensuring an adequate seal	To prevent leakage
Put form and specimen pot in specimen bag and seal	To ensure request and specimen arrive at laboratory together
Offer mouthwash/oral hygiene equipment	To maintain client comfort
Send specimen promptly to laboratory	To enable analysis of specimen. Delay in sending the specimen will invalidate the test
Document in client's notes that specimen has been obtained	To ensure consistency of care

Administration of oxygen

Oxygen (O_2) is administered as a corrective treatment for conditions resulting in hypoxia (low level of oxygen in the blood). Oxygen is classed as a medication and must be prescribed by a doctor and administered correctly to prevent over- or under-oxygenation.

Remember oxygen is NOT flammable, but it does aid combustion. Patients and visitors should therefore be educated about the increased risk of fire and the precautions necessary to reduce this risk when supplementary oxygen is in use (see 'General considerations' below).

Oxygen must only be administered at the rate and percentage prescribed, as over-oxygenation can be dangerous for some individuals, particularly those with chronic lung disease who are retaining carbon dioxide, and infants, where there is also a risk of retinopathy.

Equipment

The equipment required consists of a mask or nasal cannula that enables the administration of the prescribed dose (percentage) (see Table 1.1); connection tubing; flow meter; wall or cylinder oxygen supply (oxygen cylinders are black with a white collar); and a humidifier with sterile water if required. The procedures and rationales are given below.

Procedure	Rationale
Explain procedure, addressing health and safety precautions, and ensure adequate understanding	To promote client co-operation and safety
Wash hands following correct procedure	To prevent cross-infection
Assemble equipment - For rates of 40% and over, humidification (moistening of the oxygen prior to it reaching the client) is essential	To prevent dehydration of mucous membranes
Set flow meter to prescribed rate, e.g. 2 litres per minute	To prevent over/under-oxygenation. **NB** It may be necessary to monitor the client's oxygen saturation rate (O_2Sat) to ensure this, particularly clients with chronic lung disease, where there is a risk of apnoea, and babies, where the O_2Sat rate should not be allowed to rise above 99% as there is a significant risk of brain damage
Assist client to position mask (if mouth breathing) or nasal cannula correctly, ensuring a comfortable but not too tight a fit	To facilitate optimum administration, promote patient comfort and reduce the potential for pressure sores
Clients undergoing prolonged oxygen therapy will require monitoring of mucosa and frequent mouth/nasal care (minimum 2 hourly, see Chapter 3)	To reduce the risk of dehydration and promote patient comfort

Procedure	Rationale
Encourage client to relieve the pressure of the mask or cannula from the face, nares and ears hourly as appropriate	To reduce the potential for pressure sores
Continue to monitor the client and promptly report any change in condition	To ensure compliance and to optimize treatment
Update nursing care plan	To ensure consistency in care delivery

Table 1.1 Methods of oxygen administration

Type of system	Flow rate (l/min)	Approximate oxygen concentration delivered	Benefits	Problems	Nursing care
LOW FLOW SYSTEMS					
Nasal cannula	1 2 3 4 5 6	22-24% 26-28% 28-30% 32-36% 36-40% 40-44%	Comfortable. Convenient. Allows client to talk and eat. Mouth breathing will not affect the concentration of delivered oxygen	Unable to deliver concentrations above 44%. Assumes an adequate breathing pattern	Keep nosepieces clean. Evaluate for pressure sores over ears, cheeks and nares. Lubricate nasal prongs
Simple face mask	5-6 6-7 7-8	40% 50% 60%	If client's ventilatory needs exceed the flow of gas, the holes at the side permit air entry. Can deliver higher levels of oxygen than nasal cannulae	Mask needs to be removed for eating and drinking. Tight seal can cause facial irritation. May cause anxiety in some people, especially children. Can feel hot and claustrophobic	Mask should be removed and cleaned several times a day. Powdering of face may make mask more comfortable. Good oral hygiene essential
HIGH FLOW SYSTEMS					
Venturi mask	3 6 8	24% 26% 28% 30% 35% 40% 50%	This mask is designed to deliver accurate concentrations of oxygen	May irritate the face and skin. Interferes with eating and drinking. Tight seal needed, increasing risk to skin integrity. Condensation may collect within the system	As with simple face mask. Ensure tight fit at all times
Oxygen hood	10-12	Oxygen analyser usually fitted	Covers head leaving body free. Ideal for infants	Can feel claustrophobic	Monitoring of eye condition crucial
Tracheostomy mask			If client's needs exceed the flow of gas, the holes at the side permit air entry	Tight seal can cause irritation and soreness	Mask should be removed and cleaned several times a day

Humidification

Humidity is the amount of water vapour present in a gaseous environment. Normally, the air travelling through the airways is warmed, moistened and filtered by cells in the nasopharynx and down the airways, so that by the time it reaches the alveoli it is fully saturated at a temperature of 37°C.

This humidification is necessary to compensate for the normal loss of water from the respiratory tract. If the humidification apparatus of the body is impaired (as with disease and/or dehydration), alternative methods of humidification may need to be considered.

Oxygen therapy will further compound these problems, causing further dehydration of mucous membranes and pulmonary secretions. As a rule of thumb oxygen usually requires humidifying if delivered at or above 40 per cent or if therapy is prolonged, that is, for more than four hours. If in doubt seek advice.

External humidification is, however, essential when oxygen therapy is being delivered to a patient whose physiological humidification has been bypassed by an endotracheal tube or tracheostomy tube.

Methods of humidification

There are many devices that can be used to supply humidification (see Table 1.2). The best of these will fulfil the following requirements:

1 The inspired gas must be delivered to the trachea at a room temperature of 32-36°C and should have a water content of 33-43 g/M^3.
2 The set temperature should remain constant; large ranges of flow should not affect humidification and temperature.
3 The device should have a safety and alarm system to guard against overheating, over-hydration and electric shocks.
4 It is important that the appliance should not increase resistance or affect the compliance to respiration.
5 It is essential that whichever device is selected, wide-bore tubing, that is, tubing with a wide internal diameter (sometimes referred to as elephant tubing), must be used.

General considerations of oxygen administration

1 Oxygen is an odourless, tasteless, colourless, transparent gas that is slightly heavier than air.
2 Oxygen supports combustion, therefore there is always a danger of fire when oxygen is being used.
   The following safety measures should be remembered:
   (a) Oil or grease around oxygen connections should be avoided.

(b) Alcohol, ether and other inflammatory liquids should be used with caution in the vicinity of oxygen.
(c) No electrical device must be used in or near an oxygen tent.
(d) Oxygen cylinders should be kept secure in an upright position and away from heat.
(e) There must be no smoking in the vicinity of oxygen.
(f) A fire extinguisher should be readily available and *all* staff have a responsibility to be competent in its use.

Table 1.2 Devices for humidification

Device	Use	Benefits	Problems
Condensers (Swedish nose)	Perform function of nasopharynx	Retain heat and water from expired air and return to inspired air	Heated humidifiers may be preferable for long-term use
Cold water bubble humidifiers	Deliver partially humid-ified oxygen	Achieve about 50% humidity	Inefficient
Water bath humidifiers	Deliver adequately humidified oxygen	Achieve about 100% humidity	Overheating may damage trachea. Efficiency can alter with flow rate/surface area and water temperature. Condensation and collection of water in delivery tubes. Micro-contamination of stagnant water possible
Aerosol generators	Provide micro-droplets of water suspended in the gas	Can achieve highly saturated gas. Device not governed by temperature	

Artificial respiration (rescue breathing)

In clients who have stopped breathing it is essential to give mouth-to-mouth, mouth-to-nose, or mouth-to-mouth-and-nose ventilation until normal respiratory function is restored. If the client's breathing and pulse have stopped cardiopulmonary resuscitation (CPR) **must** be initiated immediately. The procedures and rationales are given below.

ADULT	Procedure	Rationale
	Check airway is clear as previously described and remove any obvious obstruction	To facilitate respirations
	Check for breathing	It is dangerous to perform artificial ventilation on someone who has normal respiratory function
	Look for chest movements	Absence of a rise and fall of the chest indicates absence of respiratory function
	Listen for breath sounds	Absence indicates absence of respiratory function
	Feel for breath on your cheek	Absence of warm blowing from the mouth indicates absence of respiratory function
	Look, listen and feel for no more than 10 seconds. If the client is not breathing get help, then:	To ensure that respiration has ceased
	Lie client flat on their back (supine)	To facilitate access to airways
	Tilt head and lift chin (see Figure 1.1a)	To ensure tongue is lifted away from the throat, ensuring a clear airway
	Pinch the client's nose	To ensure exhaled air is forced into the lungs and not out of the nasal passages
	Take a deep breath	To ensure lungs are expanded with sufficient air to ventilate the client
	Place your lips securely around the client's mouth	To ensure a good seal and prevent leakage of air
	Blow into the client's mouth for approximately 2 seconds, watching for the chest rising	Expelled air will enter client's lung fields, providing some oxygen. The chest rising indicates that air has entered the lung fields and not the stomach
	If chest fails to rise recheck position and airway	Air may be entering the stomach as opposed to the lung fields
	Remove your lips from the client's mouth and allow the chest to fall	To facilitate exhalation
	Repeat at a rate of 10 breaths per minute until the client starts to breathe on their own	To sustain respiratory function
	Place client in recovery position once normal respiratory function is restored	To maintain client safety
	Seek assistance	To enable investigation and treatment of cause

CHILD	Procedure	Rationale
	Check airway is clear as described above	To facilitate respirations
	Check for breathing	It is dangerous to perform artificial ventilation on someone who has normal respiratory function
	Look for chest movements	Absence of a rise and fall of the chest indicates absence of respiratory function
	Listen for breath sounds	Absence indicates absence of respiratory function
	Feel for breath on your cheek	Absence of warm blowing from the mouth indicates absence of respiratory function
	Look, listen and feel for no more than 10 seconds. If the client is not breathing get help, then:	To ensure that respiration has ceased
	Lie client flat on their back	To facilitate access to airways
	Tilt head and lift chin into 'sniffing' position (see Figure 1.2a)	To ensure tongue is lifted away from the throat, ensuring a clear airway
	Pinch the child's nose (unless mouth-to-mouth-and-nose ventilation is to be used)	To ensure exhaled air is forced into the lungs and not out of the nasal passages
	Place your lips securely around the child's mouth (or mouth and nose in a small child)	To ensure a good seal and prevent leakage of air
	Blow into the child's mouth for approximately 1-1.5 seconds, watching for the chest rising	Expelled air will enter child's lung fields, providing some oxygen. The chest rising indicates that air has entered the lung fields and not the stomach
	If chest fails to rise recheck position and airway	Air may be entering the stomach as opposed to the lung fields
	Remove your lips from the child's mouth and allow the chest to fall	To facilitate exhalation
	Repeat at a rate of 20 breaths per minute until the child starts to breathe on their own	To sustain respiratory function
	Assist the child to find a comfortable position once normal respiratory function is restored	A child will often find the best position to maintain their airway and should not be forced into position which is less than comfortable
	Seek assistance	To enable investigation and treatment of cause

INFANT	Procedure	Rationale
	Check airway is clear as described above	To facilitate respirations
	Check for breathing	It is dangerous to perform artificial ventilation on someone who has normal respiratory function
	Look for chest movements	Absence of a rise and fall of the chest indicates absence of respiratory function
	Listen for breath sounds	Absence indicates absence of respiratory function
	Feel for breath on your cheek	Absence of warm blowing from the mouth indicates absence of respiratory function
	Look, listen and feel for no more than 10 seconds. If the client is not breathing get help, then:	To ensure that respiration has ceased
	Lie infant flat on their back	To facilitate access to airways
	Tilt head and lift chin into neutral position (see Figure 1.3)	To ensure a clear airway
	Place your lips securely around the infant's mouth and nose	To ensure a good seal and prevent leakage of air
	Blow into the infant's mouth for approximately 1-1.5 seconds, watching for the chest rising	Expelled air will enter infant's lung fields, providing some oxygen. The chest rising indicates that air has entered the lung fields and not the stomach
	If chest fails to rise recheck position and airway	Air may be entering the stomach as opposed to the lung fields
	Remove your lips from the infant's mouth and allow the chest to fall	To facilitate exhalation
	Repeat at a rate of 20 breaths per minute until the infant starts to breathe on their own	To sustain respiratory function
	Assist the infant to find a comfortable position once normal respiratory function is restored	An infant will often find the best position to maintain their airway and should not be forced into position which is less than comfortable
	Seek assistance	To enable investigation and treatment of cause

References and further reading

Allen D (1989) Making sense of oxygen delivery. Nursing Times 85(18): 40–42.

Anonymous (1994) Guidelines for paediatric life support. Paediatric Life Support Working Party of the European Resuscitation Council. Resuscitation 27: 91–105.

Ashurst S (1995) Oxygen therapy. British Journal of Nursing 4(9): 508–515.

Asthma Training Centre (1997) Asthma Training Centre Learning Package. Stratford-upon-Avon: ATC.

Baillie L (Ed.) (2001) Developing Practical Nursing Skills. London: Arnold.

Bellamy D, Bellamy G (1990) Peak flow monitoring. Practice Nurse 2: 406–408.

British Medical Association (1997) Advanced Paediatric Life Support (UK) Instructors Manual. London: BMA.

Boylan A, Brown P (1985) Respirations. Nursing Times 81: 35–38.

Campbell S, Glasper EA (1995) Whaley and Wong's Children's Nursing. London: Mosby.

Carter B, Dearmun A (Eds) (1995) Child Health Care Nursing: Concepts, Theory and Practice. Oxford: Blackwell Science.

Clark JE (1990) Clinical Nursing Manual. Hemel Hempstead: Prentice Hall.

Dunn L, Chisholm H (1998) Oxygen therapy. Nursing Standard 13(7): 57–60.

Ellis JR, Nowlis EA, Bentz PM (1996) Modules for Basic Nursing Skills, 6th edn. Philadelphia, PA: Lippencott.

English I (1994) Oxygen mask or nasal catheter – an analysis. Nursing Standard 8(26): 27–30.

ERC (2000) Guidelines 2000 for Adult and Paediatric Basic Life Support. London: European Resuscitation Council.

Fell H, Boehm M (1998) Easing the discomfort of oxygen therapy. Nursing Times 94(38): 56–58.

Grey A (1995) Breathless. Nursing Times 19(27): 46–47.

Hull D, Hohnstone D (1999) Essential Paediatrics, 4th edn. Edinburgh: Churchill Livingstone.

Jones S (1997) Oxygen therapy. Community Nursing 3: 234.

Kendsrick A, Smith E (1992) Respiratory measurements 2: Simple measurement of lung function. Professional Nurse 7(1): 748–754.

Mackway-Jones K, Molyneux E, Phillips B, Wieteska S (2001) Advanced Paediatric Life Support: The Practical Approach, 3rd edn. London: BMJ Books.

Macleod JA (1992) Collecting specimens for the laboratory tests. Nursing Standard 6(20): 36–37.

Mallett J, Dougherty L (2000) The Royal Marsden Hospital: Manual of Clinical Nursing Procedures, 5th edn. London: Blackwell Science.

Matthews P (1997) Using a peak flow meter. Nursing 97: 57–59.

Mims CA, Playfair J, Roitt I, et al (1993) Medical Microbiology. St Louis, MI: CV Mosby.

Resuscitation Council UK (2000a) Basic Life Support Resuscitation Guidelines 2000, http://www.resus.org.uk. (Accessed 20 March 2003).

Resuscitation Council UK (2000b) Paediatric Basic Life Support Resuscitation Guidelines 2000, http://www.resus.org.uk. (Accessed 20 March 2003).

Roper N, Logan WW, Tierney A (1996) The Elements of Nursing, 4th edn. Edinburgh: Churchill Livingstone.

Roper N, Logan WW, Tierney A (2000) The Roper-Logan-Tierney Model of Nursing: The Activities of Living Model. Edinburgh: Churchill Livingstone.

Semple M, Elley K (1998) Collecting a sputum specimen. Nursing Times 94(48): insert: Practical Procedures No. 19 (2–8 December).

Timby B (1989) Clinical Nursing Procedures. Philadelphia, PA: JB Lippincott.

Torrance C, Hale N (1992) Respiratory observations. Surgical Nurse 5(3): 22–25.

Walsh M (2002) Watson's Clinical Nursing and Related Sciences, 6th edn. London: Ballière Tindall.

Zideman D, Zaritsky A, Waldemar MD, et al (2001) Airways in pediatric and newborn resuscitation. Annals of Emergency Medicine 37(4): S126–S136.

Chapter 2

Mobilizing

Samantha Athorn and Penelope Ann Hilton

Introduction

Motor function and the ability to move involve all parts of the motor nervous system. Injury, malformation or disease to any part of this system will therefore affect the individual's ability to move. The motor nervous system includes:

- *The central nervous system (CNS)*: this is composed of the brain and spinal cord and is responsible for initiating and co-ordinating movement.
- *The peripheral nervous system*: this consists of nerve pairings, which radiate to the various parts of the body from the CNS. These pairs of nerves send messages to and from the brain.
- *Muscles, ligaments and tendons*: these are located throughout the body and respond to sensory information. Muscles use the pulling forces of contraction and work in antagonistic pairs, that is, they oppose each other.
- *The skeleton*: this provides a system of support with a variety of joints that enable a wide range of movements.
- *The spine and discs*: these form a significant part of the skeleton and have particular notable functions:

Functions of the spine	Functions of the discs
Protects the spinal cord	Act as shock absorbers
Provides central support and stability	Vertebral spacers
Enables a range of movement	Reduction of friction
Ligament and muscle attachment	Limit over-extension/movement

It is therefore clear that the skills of movement are complex and involve both conscious decision-making and other subconscious changes such as reflex actions; together these enable us to move and complete everyday tasks such as cleansing, dressing and eliminating, as well as walking.

As individuals, the ability to move and the range of movements we can undertake are learnt and developed from those basic functions present at birth. The degree of movement, and thus ability to function in all aspects of life, are unique to the individual. This ability can be affected by many factors – not just by injury, malformation and disease.

The factors that may affect mobility may be:

- *Physical* arising from altered structures, function or processes of movement, for instance weakness arising from conditions such as anaemia, neurological or muscular impairment, or fractures.
- *Psychological* including depression, fear and anxiety (particularly in older people) and altered body image, for example stroke or amputation.
- *Pain* including that affecting general joint/muscle movement.
- *Environmental/social* such as poor housing, obstructions and other hazards, and social isolation.
- *Politico-economic* for example lack of finances for aids, adaptations and employed help.

Some of the risks associated with immobility include:

- *Physical*
  increased risk of deep vein thrombosis
  increased risk to skin integrity and pressure sore development
  increased risk of development of chest infection/pneumonia
  increased risk of urinary tract infection
  increased risk of constipation
  decreased joint and muscle movement resulting in muscle atrophy and
    increase in generalized aches and pains, for example drop foot and
    contractures

- *Psychological*
  anxiety
  depression
  loss of independence
  loss of self-esteem

- *Sociocultural*
  increased social isolation and loneliness
  increased inability to function independently in society
  loss of social identity
  forced changes in social activities

- *Politico-economic*
  loss of income arising from an inability to work

- *Environmental*
  forced changes in housing or living arrangements.

These are just some of the many possible consequences of prolonged immobility. Optimizing clients' mobility is therefore an essential nursing skill and should be undertaken in collaboration with other members of the multidisciplinary team (MDT), which includes physiotherapists, social workers, occupational therapists, remedial gymnasts, appliance officers, as well as the client, carers and medical staff.

The remainder of this chapter gives the common terminology associated with the activity of mobilizing; some of the simple principles of safe manual handling; points to consider when assessing an individual's ability to mobilize; moving; handling and positioning clients; care of an individual who is falling; and care following a fall. The chapter concludes with references and further reading.

Common terminology

Abduction	Moving away from the median line
Adduction	Moving towards the median line
Assistance	Requires help with tasks, but is also able to undertake some parts of task independently
Biomechanics	Looks at effects of movement and normal patterns of movements
Circumduction	Moving through a circle, in combination
Contraction	Shortening or drawing together
Contractures	Deformity caused by shortening of muscles, tendons and ligaments
Dependent	Unable to help, needs full assistance to achieve task
Disability	Any restriction or lack of ability to perform an activity with the socially accepted norms
Dorsal	Relating to the back
Dorsiflexion	Bending of the foot and toes upwards
Ergonomics	Looks at effective use of energy in relation to efficient movement
Eversion	Turning outwards
Extension	Straightening
External rotation	Rolling outwards
Flexion	Bending
Handicap	A disadvantage for a given individual resulting from an impairment or disability that prevents fulfilment of a role in what is perceived as the normal manner
Hemiparesis	Weakness/paralysis on one side of the body
Hemiplegia	Paralysis on one side of the body
Impairment	Any loss or abnormality of physical or psychological function
Independent	Needs no assistance with task
Internal rotation	Rolling inwards

Inversion	Turning inwards
Paralysis	Impairment or loss of motor function
Plantar	Related to the sole of the foot, as in plantar reflex
Position	Posture or placement
Pronation	Turning the palm of the hand downwards
Prone	Lying face downwards
Quadriplegia	Paralysis of all four limbs
Recumbent	Lying down in the dorsal position, i.e. on the back
Reflex	An involuntary action
Semi-prone	Lying on one side
Semi-recumbent	Lying down in the dorsal position with a pillow under the head
Supervision	Needs verbal encouragement and observation with the task
Supination	Turning upwards
Supine	Lying on the back with the face upwards
30° tilt	Lying on the back with the skeleton tilted 30° to relieve pressure on the sacrum

Assessing an individual's ability to mobilize

Motor function and the ability to move can impact on both quality and quantity of life. A full assessment of the person's ability to mobilize should therefore be undertaken on admission/arrival and at all other times when changes to the individual's abilities occur. Alongside this, movement and handling assessments should be undertaken to optimize the individual's mobility, whilst at the same time caring for oneself. An example of an assessment form is given in Figure 2.1. Where a mobility deficit is identified assessment of pressure sore risk is also vital. Figure 2.2 gives an example of a pressure risk assessment tool.

Remember that assessment of mobility is only part of a holistic nursing assessment and should not be undertaken in isolation without reference to or consideration of the client's other activities of living.

Specific points to consider when assessing an individual's ability to mobilize include:

- *Physical*
  Does the client have a fully functioning motor nervous system?
  Is there any alteration in structure, function or processes?
  Is the client able to undertake a full range of movements?
  Are there any obvious fractures, swelling or other signs of injury?
  Does the client have any pain inhibiting mobility?
  Is this related to any specific movements?
  Does the client have any reduced (or absence of) feeling or any strange or unusual sensations such as tingling in the fingers or toes?

Figure 2.1 Example of a client moving and handling assessment form

Client Details:

Date of Assessment:

Assessed by:

Designation:

Part 1: LOAD/INDIVIDUAL CAPABILITIES

Weaknesses/Disabilities

Weight .... kgs

Height .... cms

Handling Constraints (e.g. pain, level of motivation, language barriers)

Client Handling Behaviours

Client's Perceived
Actual/Potential Problems (Circle)

Co-operative	
Loss of Confidence	
Unpredictable	
Loss of Motivation	
History of Falling	
Unco-operative	

Standing	Actual/Potential
Sitting	Actual/Potential
Walking	Actual/Potential
Transferring	Actual/Potential
Toileting	Actual/Potential
Climbing Stairs	Actual/Potential

Mobility aids normally used   Y/N

Wheelchair	Prosthesis (state which):
Walking Stick	
Walking Frame	
Crutches	Other:
Adapted Footwear	
Splint(s)	

Part 2: Environment

	Yes	No	Remedial Action Taken
Environment conducive to care?			
Non-slip floor surface?			
Seating appropriate?			
Bed appropriate?			
Proximity to toilet appropriate?			

Figure 2.1 Example of a client moving and handling assessment form

Part 3: Tasks

Task	Independent	Needs assistance x 1	Needs assistance x 2	Manoeuvre required (state which)	Aids required (state which)	Type/Level of patient involvement
Standing						
Sitting up in chair						
Sitting up in bed						
Turning left to right						
Turning right to left						
Moving up the bed						
Transfer bed to chair						
Transfer bed to wheelchair						
Transfer bed to trolley						
Transfer chair to chair						
Walking						
Bathing						
Dressing						
Toileting						
Climbing stairs						

Any Additional Problems

Referrals

Moving & Handling Co-ordinator	Yes/No	Date:
Physiotherapist	Yes/No	Date:
Occupational Therapist	Yes/No	Date:
Social Worker	Yes/No	Date:
Other (please specify)	Yes/No	Date:

Signature: .... **Print Name:** ....

Figure 2.2 Example of Pressure Risk Assessment Tool

Guidelines for Completing Assessment Chart   **Client's Name:**

1. Complete initial assessment for all patients within 2 hours of admission
2. Update Waterlow Score as per patient needs (minimum weekly)   **Unit No.:**
3. If sores present: grade, document, instigate appropriate care plan, and refer to Tissue Viability Nurse   **Ward:**

10+ AT RISK   **15+ HIGH RISK**   **20+ VERY HIGH RISK**   **Audit Date:**

Date	Month															
Time																
BUILD/WEIGHT FOR HEIGHT	Average Above average Obese Below average	0 1 2 3														
CONTINENCE	Complete/Catheter Occasional incontinence Faecal incontinence Doubly incontinent	0 1 2 3														
SKIN TYPE	Healthy Tissue paper Dry Oedematous Clammy Discoloured Broken spot	0 1 1 1 1 2 3														
MOBILITY	Fully Restless/Fidgety Apathetic Restricted Inert/Traction Chair bound	0 1 2 3 4 5														
SEX/AGE	Male Female 14-49 50-64 65-74 75-80 > 81	1 2 1 2 3 4 5														
APPETITE	Average Poor NG Tube/Fluid only Anorexic/NBM	0 1 2 3														
TISSUE MALNUTRITION	Terminal cachexia Cardiac failure Peripheral vascular disease Anaemia Smoking	8 5 5 2 1														
NEURO	Diabetes, CVA, MS, Paraplegia	4/6														
SURGERY	Orthopaedic/Below Waist/ Spinal. > 2 hrs on table*	5 5														
MEDICATION	Anti-inflammatory drugs, high dose steroids, cytotoxics	4														
NURSE INITIALS																

*up to 48 hrs post operative

Figure 2.2 Example of Pressure Risk Assessment Tool

NURSING MANAGEMENT

Waterlow Assessment Score

< 10 (Low Risk)
☐ Assess patient's skin condition weekly or if condition changes
☐ Record score in care records
☐ Educate patient to relieve own pressure
☐ Complete movement plan

10+ (Low-Medium Risk)
☐ Assess patient's skin condition daily
☐ Record score in care records daily
☐ Educate patient to relieve own pressure
☐ Complete movement plan
☐ Ensure pressure-reducing foam mattress or pressure-reducing mattress overlay in situ at all times

15+ (Medium-High Risk)
☐ Assess patient's skin condition every shift
☐ Record score in care records daily unless score changes; if so document accordingly
☐ Educate patient to relieve own pressure areas
☐ Discuss, with patient, moving and handling techniques
☐ Ensure dynamic pressure-relieving mattress in situ at all times when in bed as per local policy and pressure-relieving cushion in situ when using chair

20+ (High-Very High Risk)
☐ Turn or tilt patient on a 2-4 hourly basis and assess patient's skin condition on each occasion
☐ Record score in care records daily unless score changes; if so document accordingly
☐ Educate patient to relieve own pressure areas
☐ Discuss, with patient, moving and handling techniques
☐ Ensure dynamic pressure-relieving mattress in situ at all times when in bed as per local policy and pressure-relieving cushion in situ when using chair
☐ Refer to Tissue Viability Nurse for further advice and guidance
☐ Refer to other agencies as necessary, e.g. dietetics, physiotherapy, medics

Adapted from Waterlow (1985)

Does the client use any aids, for example wheelchair, frame, walking stick, specially adapted footwear?

Does the client have any illnesses or disorders that might affect their ability to mobilize, for example lung disease, anaemia, vertigo?

If reduced, does their limited mobility inhibit other activities, for example cleansing and dressing?

If impaired, is this likely to be temporary or permanent?

- *Psychological*
  Is the client depressed?
  Anxious?
  Frightened?
  What is their level of motivation?
  What does the client consider influences their ability to mobilize?

- *Sociocultural*
  Are they able to carry out fundamental domestic activities such as cooking, cleaning, shopping?
  Do they walk, drive, use public transport?
  What type of social activities do they undertake, for example vigorous, sedentary?
  Are they involved in any sporting activities, for example swimming, dancing?
  What is their type of employment, if any, for example manual, sedentary?
  What is their preferred style of dress?
  Does this enhance or inhibit the potential to mobilize, for example high heels, worn carpet slippers, tight-fitting trousers?

- *Environmental*
  What is their type and place of residence, for example high-rise flat, urban, rural?
  What type of terrain does the client need to negotiate?
  Is the client able to negotiate stairs?
  Is this a necessary function prior to discharge?
  What available space do they have to mobilize at home/in the care environment?
  Is this conducive to mobilizing?
  Are there any obstructions?
  Is the environment safe in which to mobilize?
  Does the client feel safe?
  Type and design of furniture: is this conducive to mobilizing?
  Will the current change of environment affect them in any way, for example further to walk to the toilet, washroom?

- *Politico-economic*
  Is the client financially independent?

Do they need assistance with the purchase of aids and adaptations?
Is there local provision for sport and social activity?
Is there adequate street lighting, safe pavements and crossings in their locality?
Is local transport accessible?
Can public buildings be easily accessed?
Are there any facilities to exercise in the locality?

- *Past history*
Does the client have a history of falls or difficulty mobilizing?
Does the client normally exercise, if so to what degree?

Moving and handling

Manual handling is defined as 'the lifting, lowering, pushing, pulling, carrying, transporting or supporting by hand or bodily force any object including a person' (Health and Safety Executive, 1992).

The emphasis for movement and handling must be to undertake an efficient movement, using a suitable and appropriate method whilst maintaining client safety and comfort. An efficient movement is one that achieves the objective by employing minimal effort to do so with the minimum of strain.

The term 'lifting' has previously been widely used to refer to movement and handling activities. However, this term has been seen to indicate the need to take the client's full weight as part of movement and handling. In recent years it has become readily apparent that to undertake such a manoeuvre is potentially dangerous for both the nurse and the client. For these reasons, 'lifting' is now considered an inappropriate term and its use to describe movement and handling activities is discouraged. Indeed the manual lifting of clients is now deemed unsafe in most institutions and is not generally recommended under any circumstances.

Care of self

Back injury is the largest single cause of long-term sickness, with reported back pain being most common in those with skilled manual, partly skilled and unskilled jobs. The true cost of back injury to industry is difficult to define.

There is now a great deal of legislation relating to manual handling, which sets out responsibilities and gives guidance for both employers and employees. The dangers of manual handling to the nurse are now well understood: 'One in four qualified nurses has taken time off with a back injury sustained at work and for some it has meant the end of their nursing career' (Disabled Living Foundation, 1994). All nurses and carers must be aware of and consider these risks and adopt safe principles of manual handling. The need for safety in practice has now been recognized as a fundamental necessity.

The UKCC (1996) stated: 'although the most important consideration must be the patient's safety and well being, this must not be at the expense of the nurse's health and safety'.

The importance of looking after one's back is vitally important, not only at work but also at all other times during the day. An injury sustained outside of work will still have the same effect on a career involving movement and handling activities as one sustained during these duties. Caring for oneself and one's back should therefore be a 24-hour responsibility and the reader is reminded that the adoption of safe movement and handling techniques outside of work is just as important as undertaking these at work. By avoiding top-heavy postures and following simple principles of safe movement and handling, it is possible to maintain a fit and healthy back and consequently look forward to a long and rewarding career.

Top-heavy posture

Top-heavy posture relates to positions where the individual is leaning slightly forwards or bending forward with the spine arched and not in its natural line. This position is often adopted unconsciously, with the individual being unaware of the fact that they are bending and arching the spine. Although immediate problems may not be felt, both short- and long-term effects and injury can occur with the recurrent use of a top-heavy posture.

Simple principles of safe manual handling

Thinking through each individual situation and applying the following simple principles when moving and handling will enable you to maintain health and safety whilst undertaking the task.

- **Assessment of the task**
  A full and comprehensive assessment should be made of the task before undertaking the move. This assessment of all aspects of the task will enable you to identify risks and hazards and to problem solve to enable the undertaking of safe manoeuvres (see the section on 'Moving inanimate objects', p. 35).

- **Maintain a stable base**
  Position the feet slightly apart, with the lead foot pointing in the direction of movement.
  Stability provided by positioning the feet in such a way will prevent loss of balance and falling or twisting during the manoeuvre.
  When moving and handling a client, for example from one bed to another, it may seem impossible to keep both feet on the floor to provide a stable base without over stretching. It is possible and the situation should be reassessed so as to ensure a stable base whilst undertaking the move. If this is difficult seek guidance from the in-house moving and handling trainer.

- **Lower the centre of gravity**
  By bending or flexing the knees slightly, the centre of gravity will be lowered. This bending of the knees will not only help the posture to be more relaxed and less taut but also provide more stability.

- **Keep the spine in line**
  The spine's natural curves should be maintained in their normal position, often referred to as 'in line', to prevent the occurrence of injury during movement and handling activities. Keeping the spine 'in line' also means avoiding top-heavy postures and positions where the spine is twisted or rotated at any point.

- **Keep the load close to your body**
  Keeping the load close to the body reduces the strain/effort involved in the manoeuvre, by having the load closer to the centre of gravity.
  It increases efficiency of the movement.
  It reduces the likelihood of injury.

- **Move your head up**
  Raising the head in an upward direction/movement when undertaking a move leads the body in its movement and helps maintain good posture throughout.

- **Holds**
  Holds used should be relaxed palm-type holds or stroking. Grasping or direct holds should not be used.
  Using indirect holds allows the hold to be released should the manoeuvre be beyond one's abilities and reduces the likelihood of injury.
  Stroking down clients' limbs to aid in their movement is gentler for the client and they are less likely to respond by suddenly withdrawing the limb, which could result in one being jerked or injured.

- **Remember individual capabilities**
  Remember to consider the individual capabilities of all concerned in the manoeuvre; this includes you and your colleagues as well as the client.

Those who have had previous injuries, or pregnant women, may be at greater risk when moving and handling.

- **Know the equipment**
  It is important to know not only what equipment is available, but also how to use it correctly and to its fullest potential. One should also be aware of the correct methods for sizing of slings/accessories to ensure these are used correctly.
  The maximum safe working load of all pieces of equipment used in the area should be known.
  Equipment should be well maintained and serviced regularly. Do not use if faulty and ensure that faulty equipment is labelled as such and reported immediately.
  All equipment should be checked at least annually and a record kept.

- **Good communication**
  Good communication is important so that everyone involved in the manoeuvre is aware of what their responsibilities are in relation to the move, and when the manoeuvre is to take place. This will also help to ensure that the move is carried out at the correct time in an organized manner.
  Communication with the client is also vital not only to ensure their co-operation but also to maintain their trust and confidence.

- **Controlled manoeuvres**
  Remember that manoeuvres need to be controlled and taken in stages if necessary to avoid over-stretching for those undertaking the move and to avoid discomfort or fear for the client.

- **Wear appropriate clothing and footwear**
  Wearing correctly fitting and appropriate clothing will enable free movement without being restricted.
  Correct footwear will ensure good stability and grip and thus prevent over-balancing or slipping.

- **Avoid manual handling**
  Manual handling, that is, physically moving objects or persons, should be avoided if at all possible.

Remembering these principles and being able to apply them in the variety of movement and handling tasks undertaken both in the workplace and in everyday life will enable problem solving and the identification of safe solutions in respect of movement and handling.

Adopting these principles will provide a more flexible approach to manual handling than learning a specific move for a specific situation, where in real life other factors involved often make such specific manoeuvres learnt unsuitable or unachievable in the practice setting.

Legally, every employer must ensure that his or her employees receive adequate health and safety training including manual handling training (see Chapter 4). This training should be repeated periodically where appropriate, usually annually, and adapted to take into account any new or changed risks. Therefore, any changes made after assessing a manual handling operation should be accompanied by a degree of training. The employee is duty bound to attend these training sessions.

Assessing the task, individual capabilities, load and environment

The four crucial elements of risk assessment are: task, load, individual and environment. Assessment of these four elements is fundamental to a thorough undertaking of a risk assessment regarding any manual handling procedure.

A risk is seen as the chance of something happening that will have an impact on objectives. The consequences and likelihood of the identified risk can then be ascertained to demonstrate the level of risk involved in the manoeuvre.

The following assessments of these four crucial elements should be undertaken to identify the risks involved, thus enabling a problem solving approach to be undertaken to reduce or remove the risks before commencing any manoeuvre in keeping with the Health and Safety at Work Act (1974).

The task

- Does this manoeuvre need to be done?
- Does the task require unusual capabilities?
- Can the client move him- or herself or can they help?
- Is the client able to comprehend your instructions?
- What equipment or moving aids are available?
- Why is the task being undertaken?
- What are the start and end points of the task – where are we going?

Does the task involve:

- holding the load away from the trunk at a distance?
- unsatisfactory posture, including twisting, stooping, or reaching upwards?
- excessive movement of the load over large vertical distances?
- risk of sudden movement or unpredictable load?
- repetitive or prolonged physical effort?
- strenuous movement of the load by pushing or pulling?
- are there sufficient rest or recovery periods?

Individual capability

- Is the handler fit for the task?
- What experience do they have?
- Are they familiar with the equipment?
- Are they pregnant?
- Have they any history of back injury?
- Are they hindered by clothing or personal protective equipment?

The load

- Is the load heavy?
- Is the load bulky or unwieldy?
- Are there difficulties in holding the load?
- Is the load unstable or likely to be unpredictable?
- Could the load be harmful?

If the load is a client:

- What is the client's diagnosis and will this affect the task?
- Can the client help?
- Is the client in pain?
- Are there other constraints such as tubes, lines or other equipment in use?
- Is the client anxious or confused?
- Are there any other factors with this individual that may affect the task?

The environment

- What space is available, or does this cause constraint?
- Can equipment, furniture or other items be moved around to create a better environment?
- Is the floor surface area safe, dry, slippery, even?
- Are the lighting conditions suitable?
- Are the temperature/conditions suitable?
- Is this a safe environment for movement and handling of clients?

A thorough assessment of all these factors and any other identified risk or hazards should always be undertaken prior to each move, and the identified risks reduced, removed or safe working practices used.

Moving inanimate objects

Whatever the object to be moved and handled, it is essential to perform a thorough assessment of risk and to follow the simple principles of safe manual handling as outlined above when undertaking any manoeuvre.

Whilst the lifting of clients is not generally recommended there will be occasions when it is necessary to lift inanimate objects. The Manual Handling Operations Regulations (Health and Safety Executive 1992) offer some numerical guidelines on acceptable weights (see Table 2.1). Lifting within these boundaries is unlikely to result in injury.

Table 2.1 The Manual Handling Operations Guidance on weight limits for lifting and lowering   (HSE, 1992)

Height object held at	Weight limit for		Weight limit for	
	Man	Woman	Man	Woman
	Object held at arm's length		Object held close in to trunk	
Full height	5 kg	3 kg	10 kg	7 kg
Shoulder height	10 kg	7 kg	20 kg	13 kg
Elbow height	15 kg	10 kg	25 kg	17 kg
Knuckle height	10 kg	7 kg	20 kg	13 kg
Mid-lower leg	5 kg	3 kg	10 kg	7 kg

However, even in these circumstances, assessment of the task should be undertaken to facilitate the reduction of risks. The regulations also state that information should be provided regarding the weight of loads. Sometimes this information is not always available. Attempts to gauge the weight of an object by its size or appearance alone have been shown to be wholly inaccurate; therefore if unsure don't guess – seek help.

It is important to remember that the figures given in Table 2.1 are provided as guideline figures, and should always be used in conjunction with the risk assessment of:

- task
- individual capabilities
- load
- environment.

The principles of safe manual handling should always be followed:

- spine in line
- stable base

- load kept close to the body
- head moving up and leading
- only manually handling if necessary
- knowing and using appropriate equipment/aids
- correct holds
- lowered centre of gravity
- controlled manoeuvre
- good communication.

Moving and positioning clients

Prior to moving, handling and positioning of any clients, a movement and handling risk assessment should be undertaken (see above) to fulfil the Health and Safety Regulations concerning the manual handling of loads. The Manual Handling Operations Regulations (1992) state that when hazardous manual handling tasks cannot be eliminated, a 'suitable and sufficient' written assessment should be undertaken.

In addition to undertaking a risk assessment, the handler/s should:

- follow safe principles of manual handling
- follow safe systems of practice, in accordance with training
- follow the written movement and handling risk assessment or reassess
- take care of self and colleagues' health and safety
- fully utilize appropriate equipment and moving aids provided.

When moving and positioning clients, ask the following:

- Does the move need to be undertaken – why are you undertaking the manoeuvre?
- Is there a documented movement and handling assessment and is this current or in need of updating?
- Can the client help with the manoeuvre, or undertake the manoeuvre with supervision?
- What equipment is available to help with this manoeuvre with this client and is the equipment working?
- Are the handlers trained to use the available equipment?
- Are there enough handlers available to undertake an identified manoeuvre and to use the available equipment as trained?
- What risks will the manoeuvre present?
- Which technique should be used?
- What client position are we aiming to achieve? (See Figures 2.3a–g.)

Selection of position should be based on client preference, client's condition and nursing needs.

Having asked these questions, remember the following:

- Use clear and concise communication with all handlers and the client to ensure a co-ordinated movement where all those involved are aware of their responsibilities.
- Prepare the environment, ensuring there is enough space to safely perform the manoeuvre. This may include having to move unnecessary pieces of equipment or furnishings.

Having undertaken all of this, implement the manoeuvre if safe to do so.

Always check that the client is comfortable and safe following any movement and handling procedure.

Care of an individual who is falling

When undertaking any movement and handling activity, including mobilizing of a client, the importance of undertaking a thorough assessment of the task before commencing is crucial. By undertaking a comprehensive assessment and utilizing all the information gained, it is possible to identify constraints of an activity that may result in a client falling if the manoeuvre is performed, and thus influence the decision as to whether or not to utilize such a manoeuvre.

It is much safer to prevent a client falling in the first instance than to have them fall whilst moving or mobilizing them. With good assessment, it is possible to significantly reduce the incidence of trips, slips or falls.

To aid in the assessment of clients and their ability to weight-bear a simple assessment can be performed. This involves getting the client into a seated position. The client should then be asked to raise the lower part of their legs from the knee downwards, so that the legs are straight. The ability to successfully accomplish this will indicate whether or not the client is likely to be able to weight-bear.

If a client does fall, this can have a detrimental effect not only on them, but also on their family and indeed those caring for the client. The client may be physically injured during the fall, which may result in their ability to mobilize being reduced, with the concomitant risks. There may be subsequent loss of confidence in their own abilities to mobilize, and they may suffer from heightened anxieties and fear when people are trying to help them mobilize or move them in future. Relatives of the client who has fallen may display feelings of anxiety, anger or concern that this has happened, this being particularly, but not necessarily, more likely if physical harm has actually occurred to the client as a result of falling. For

Figure 2.3 Common positions used in nursing

(a) Upright

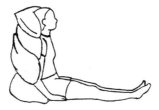

(b) Semi-prone (recovery)

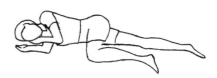

(c) Dorsal

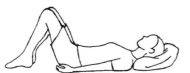

(d) Recumbent

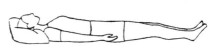

(e) Lateral

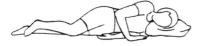

(f) Prone

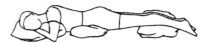

(g) Orthopnoeic

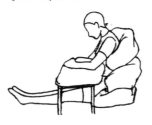

Illustrations by Sophie Kerslake

those caring for the client, there may also be feelings of anxiety. It is not uncommon for nurses to feel a sense of anger with themselves, and a great deal of responsibility, when one of their clients has fallen, and, when physical harm has occurred, these feelings are often heightened.

However, despite the best assessment and planning in the world, unfortunately, clients do occasionally fall. Remember that when things do go wrong and a client starts to fall or appears to be falling, it is by far safer for all concerned to let them fall than to attempt to catch them. The key is, whilst allowing the client to fall, to attempt to enter an element of control to the fall. This can be achieved by taking care of and cushioning the client's head and ensuring that inanimate objects such as drip stands or other pieces of equipment attached to the client do not also fall, as they have the potential to cause further injury should they hit the client.

If at all possible allow the client to fall in a more controlled way where the least possible harm will be incurred as a result of the incident.

Proceed then to treat the client who has fallen (see below), document the occurrence and undertake a post-incident risk assessment with the aim of reducing the potential for reoccurrence following local policy. It may also be prudent to inform the client's next of kin.

Care of an individual who has fallen

Care of a client who has fallen or one who has been found on the floor should include the following steps:

Procedure	Rationale
Assess the situation and approach if safe to do so	To ensure personal safety
Undertake a swift assessment of the condition of the client	To assess for life-threatening problems which require urgent medical/nursing attention
Are signs of life present?	Is this a simple fall, slip, trip or faint; or has the patient suffered a life-threatening event, e.g. cardiac arrest, resulting in their being found on the floor

Procedure	Rationale
• Is the client conscious?	If life signs are not present, cardiopulmonary resuscitation should be commenced (see Chapter 4)
• How does the client appear: pale, clammy, cyanosed? • Are they breathing? • Does the client have a pulse?	
Make the client comfortable by: • Placing a pillow under their head if appropriate. If injury to the neck is suspected this should not be undertaken • Maintaining the client's dignity	To keep the client as comfortable as possible until it is safe to move them, whilst maintaining their safety and preventing them from further harm
Get help, both medical and nursing	The client should have a medical assessment performed prior to attempting to move them from the floor to ensure that they are safe to be moved without causing further harm or injury. The help of both medical and nursing staff will ensure that identified injuries can be treated promptly, whilst enabling a member of staff to remain with the client at all times. To move a client from the floor safely requires teamwork and cannot safely be performed alone
Following assessment treat injuries needing urgent attention, where the client has fallen, before attempting to move them	To prevent further injury or discomfort
Reassure the client and keep them informed about what is happening	To reduce anxiety and increase the likelihood of co-operation
A hoist should be used to get the client from the floor, unless they can either do this for themselves or the use of a hoist is contra-indicated	It is unsafe to lift a client from the floor manually. A hoist or stretcher hoist should always be used if at all possible
Keep the patient informed and reassure continually throughout the procedure	To reduce anxiety and increase the likelihood of co-operation
If the client is attempting to get himself or herself up from the floor and it is considered safe for them to do so, they should be encouraged to roll so that they can position themselves on their hands and knees	To encourage independence and return of confidence

Procedure	Rationale
It may then be useful to place a chair for them to lean on, before attempting to stand	To reduce the potential for postural hypotension by enabling a staged return to an upright position
Ensure before allowing them to undertake this manoeuvre that the floor is not slippery and that they are wearing appropriate footwear	To maintain a safe environment
Assess the situation and move the client using appropriate, effective manoeuvres	To enable the client to be moved safely and effectively to an area where further medical/nursing assessment and treatment can be undertaken
Promote client comfort	Following movement it is important to ensure that the client feels comfortable and safe to restore confidence
Reassess for injuries	Reassessment of injuries should be undertaken once the client is comfortable and in a safe area to identify any further injuries, which may not have been identified immediately after the initial incident
Continue to monitor the client	To ensure early detection of any changes in condition
Inform Senior Nurse, complete untoward incident/accident form in keeping with local policy	To meet health and safety legislation
Update nursing care plan and movement and handling assessments	To ensure consistency in care delivery
Inform next of kin	To aid good communications and acknowledge duty of care

References and further reading

Blows WT (2001) The Biological Basis of Nursing: Clinical Observations. London: Routledge.
Brewer S (2001) Safe and sound... the Health and Safety at Work Act. Nursing Standard 15(34): 61.
Clarke M (1979) Practical Nursing. London: Ballière Tindall.
Dimond B (2002) Enforcement of statutory duties for health and safety at work. British Journal of Nursing 11(11): 745-7.

Disabled Living Foundation (1994) Moving and Handling People Factsheet. London: Disabled Living Foundation.

European Resuscitation Council (UK) (2001) Guidance for safer handling during resuscitation in hospitals. London: European Resuscitation Council (UK).

Health and Safety Executive (1992) Manual Handling: Manual Handling Operations: Guidance on Regulations. London: HSE Books.

Health and Safety Executive (1999) Health and Safety Law – What you should Know. http://www.open.gov.uk/hse/hsehome.htm. (Accessed 21 March 2003)

Mallett J, Dougherty L (2000) Manual of Clinical Nursing Procedures, 5th edn. London: Blackwell Science.

Mandelstram M (2001a) Safe use of disability equipment and manual handling: legal aspects – part 1 disability equipment. British Journal of Occupational Therapy 64(1): 9–16.

Mandelstram M (2001b) Safe use of disability equipment and manual handling: legal aspects – part 2 manual handling. British Journal of Occupational Therapy 64(2): 73–80.

Parker LJ (1999) Managing and maintaining a safe environment in the hospital setting. British Journal of Nursing 8(16): 1053–8.

Royal College of Nursing (2000) Working well initiative, RCN Code of Practice for Patient Handling. London: Royal College of Nursing.

Royal College of Nursing (2000) Working well initiative, Introducing a Safer Patient Handling Policy. London: Royal College of Nursing.

Royal College of Nursing (1990) Equipment to save your back. Nursing Standard 4(43): 26–9.

Simon P and the National Back Pain Association (1992) In the hidden scandal. Nursing Times 88(41): 24–6.

UKCC (1996) Guidelines for Professional Practice. London: UKCC.

Walsh M (2002) Watson's Clinical Nursing and Related Sciences, 6th edn. London: Ballière Tindall.

Current legislation governing safe moving and handling

Health and Safety at Work Act (1974).

Manual Handling Operations Regulations (1992).

Management of Health and Safety at Work (1999).

Workplace (Health, Safety and Welfare) Regulations (1992).

Reporting of Injuries, Diseases and Dangerous Occurrences Regulations (1995).

Provision and Use of Work Equipment Regulations (1998).

Lifting Operations and Lifting Equipment Regulations (1998).

Health and Safety Executive Bulletins. London: HMSO.

Chapter 3

Personal cleansing and dressing

Alyson Hoyles, Penelope Ann Hilton
and Neal Seymour

Introduction

The ability to cleanse and dress is a fundamental need and involves far
more than the physical act of cleansing the skin to reduce the potential
for infection and injury. Personal cleansing and dressing is also important in promoting the psychological, social, cultural and overall
well-being of the individual. In acknowledging the importance of this
aspect of care the Department of Health have outlined seven benchmarks
for best practice, which include: individual assessment of personal and
oral hygiene needs; planning negotiated care based on a sound assessment; providing a conducive environment; ensuring that clients have
toiletries for their personal use; providing adequate levels of assistance;
providing any necessary information and education to enable clients to
maintain their individual personal hygiene needs; and finally, continuous
evaluation and reassessment of care needs (see http://www.doh.gov.uk/
essenceofcare). In order to meet these standards, this chapter gives some
of the common terminology associated with personal cleansing and
dressing. It then offers a brief insight into the structure and functions of
the skin, and gives some specific points to consider when assessing a
client's personal cleansing and dressing needs. The remainder of the
chapter includes how to make up an occupied or unoccupied bed or cot;
safe disposal of linen; assisting individuals requiring bathing; assisting
individuals with oral hygiene; eye care; facial shaving; care of the hair;
and assisting individuals to dress. The chapter concludes with references
and suggestions for further reading.

Common terminology

Canthus	The angle formed at the junction of the upper and lower eyelids
Gingivitis	Inflammation of the gums
Glossitis	Inflammation of the tongue
Halitosis	Bad breath
Healthy mouth	Clean, functional and comfortable oral cavity which is free from infection
Periodontitis	Inflammation of the gums, palate and surrounding structures
Perineum	The area of skin between the external genitalia and the anus
Personal hygiene	Physical act of cleansing the body to ensure that the skin, hair and nails are maintained in an optimum condition
Plaque	A deposit of food and bacteria on the teeth, which may produce tartar and dental caries
Oral hygiene	Effective removal of plaque and debris to ensure the structures and tissues of the mouth are kept in a healthy condition
Stomatitis	Inflammation of the mouth
Tenting	A sign of dehydration where the skin, when gently pinched, is slow to return to its normal state
Turgidity	Degree of swelling
Xerostomia	Dryness of the mouth

The skin

The skin is an important organ and has a variety of functions, including:

- protection
- control of body temperature
- excretion of sweat and sebum
- sensations of touch, heat, cold, pain and pressure
- support.

Maintaining the integrity and cleanliness of the skin is therefore essential to the maintenance and promotion of health.

The skin is made up of three layers:

1 The epidermis or outer coating of the skin – cells on the surface are continually being rubbed off and replaced by new ones. Hairs and sweat glands form part of the epidermis, and the ducts of sebaceous glands pass through this layer.
2 The dermis is a thicker layer – it is tough and elastic and contains blood vessels, nerve fibres, lymph vessels, sweat and sebaceous glands.
3 The subcutaneous layer contains fat cells and provides heat regulation for the body.

The factors that may affect cleansing and dressing may be:

- *physical* arising from alterations in the structure or functions of the skin, motor or sensory deficits of the musculo-skeletal system, presence of wounds, drains, level of hearing, vision, shortness of breath
- *psychological* such as safety, self-esteem, personal space, self-image, privacy, motivation
- *sociocultural*, for example family influences, peers, groups, routines, societal standards, religious beliefs, gender
- *environmental* including facilities available, temperature, climate, time of day
- *politico-economic*, for example lack of finances, hot water, adequate resources and occupation.

Assessing an individual's ability to cleanse and dress

Remember that assessment of cleansing and dressing is only part of a holistic nursing assessment and should not be undertaken in isolation without reference to or consideration of the client's other activities of living.

Specific points to consider when assessing an individual's ability to cleanse and dress include:

- *Physical*
  Is the client able to cleanse and dress themselves independently?
  What is their stage of development?
  Do they have any changes in their physical structures, functions or processes impeding their ability to maintain personal hygiene?
  Do they have any changes in their physical structures, functions or processes impeding their ability to dress?
  Is their skin clean, intact and healthy?
  Any bruises, scars, blemishes or alteration in colour?
  Is the skin dry or moist?
  Any signs of dehydration, for example tenting or loss of elasticity?
  Are the nails clean, short and well groomed?
  Is the mouth moist and healthy?
  Are the teeth intact and well tended? Does the client wear dentures? What is their normal dental cleansing routine?
  Is the hair clean and well groomed? Are there any signs of head lice or dandruff? What is the client's normal routine?
  What is their mode of dress and is this appropriate?
  Do they have any specific requirements related to menstruation?

If male, does the client shave and if so what is their preferred method? Can this be facilitated?

Does the client have any allergies to soap, perfumes or powders?

- *Psychological*

  Are there any gender related issues, for example male client requesting a male nurse for intimate care and vice versa.

  Is the client anxious or worried about any issues related to cleansing and dressing, for example does not like to be seen without their dentures in or without their wig or make-up?

  Is the client depressed or lacking in motivation to maintain personal hygiene?

  Do they lack knowledge or skills related to maintaining cleansing and dressing, for example infection control?

- *Sociocultural*

  What are the client's values and beliefs surrounding cleansing and dressing?

  Does the client have any specific religious or cultural rituals they need or wish to follow prior to, during or following bathing (for example Muslims are expected to bathe under free-flowing water)?

  Does the client have any specific religious or cultural needs surrounding dress (for example Sikhs do not generally remove their turbans in the presence of others)?

  Are there any specific issues surrounding modesty and dignity?

  What are the client's normal routines?

- *Environmental*

  Does the client prefer a wash, bath or shower?

  Do they have adequate facilities at home for cleansing self and clothing, for example hot water, washing machine, laundrette near by?

  Is the environment conducive to personal cleansing and dressing, for example too hot/cold, public/private?

- *Politico-economic*

  Are there any financial issues, for example lack of money for clothing, heating, facilities?

  Do they use expensive toiletries, perfumes, lotions or potions?

  Can they afford cleansing materials?

Making a bed or cot

Making a bed/cot provides a clean and comfortable environment for the client as well as reducing the risk of cross-infection. It should be performed based on the individual's needs and preferences.

Equipment

Clean linen (sheets, pillowcases, blankets/duvet cover, counterpane) and a linen skip are required. The procedures and rationales are given below.

Procedure	Rationale
Plan the timing of this activity (For speed and efficacy, two staff should perform this activity, if possible)	To limit/reduce disturbance, flow of micro-organisms in the air when other activities are occurring. To fit in with client activity
Wear apron, wash hands	Prevents cross-infection. Only wear gloves if in contact with body secretions
Prepare the environment around the bed/cot	Safety for nurse
Ensure bed brakes are on	Client/nurse safety
Raise bed to an appropriate height	Reduce the risk of back injury. Nurse safety
Keep clean and dirty linen separate	Reduce the risk of cross-infection
Strip bed onto bed stripper and/or chair at the base of the bed/cot with minimal movement of bedclothes, removing each item separately	Reduces airflow and circulating organisms. To prevent items such as spectacles being sent to the laundry in error
Fold soiled linen inwards. Hold away from apron and place immediately in linen skip. Do not drop bedding on the floor	Reduces transmission of micro-organisms and risk of cross-infection
Check the mattress for wear and tear and replace if necessary	Client comfort and infection control
If soiled, clean with soap and water	Infection control
Place bottom sheet on the mattress. Open out the sheet ensuring equal amounts of material at top, bottom and sides to tuck in	To reduce slippage of sheets and potential for creasing
Ensuring sheet is flat, smooth and crease-free, make a small pleat at the foot end prior to tucking in	To increase client comfort, and to reduce the risk of pressure sores and possibility of plantar flexion
Tuck in at the base of the bed/cot, leaving sheet open at the top	To reduce slippage
Add blanket/counterpane/duvet in the same manner, according to client needs/wishes	Client comfort

Procedure	Rationale
Once complete, fold top sheet over blanket/counterpane/duvet	To promote easier access for client
Change pillowcases as required and arrange to suit client needs/wishes	Client comfort
Lower bed to suitable height for client/child and ensure bed brakes are on	To promote client safety and ease of access
Replace equipment including call button within client's reach	To promote client safety
Remove linen skip/equipment and leave area clean and tidy	To prevent cross-infection
Remove apron and wash hands	To prevent cross-infection

Changing linen on an occupied bed or cot

Making a bed or cot provides a clean and comfortable environment as well as reducing the risk of cross-infection. It should be performed on the basis of the individual's needs and preferences. Clean sheets, pillowcases, linen skip, blankets/duvet cover and counterpane are required. The procedures and rationales are given below.

Procedure	Rationale
Two nurses/carers	To ensure client safety and prevent injury to staff
Explain the procedure to the client and seek their co-operation if possible	To promote informed consent
Apply apron and wash hands	To reduce the risk of cross-infection
Plan the timing of this activity taking into account the client's needs and wishes	To reduce the risk of cross-infection within area and minimize disturbance of airflow. Meet client wishes
Draw curtains around client bed/cot. Raise bed. Remove cot sides/restraint. Safely secure drips, drain and catheters	Preserve privacy of client, care of access
Strip counterpane/duvet/blankets as above, but leaving client covered with top sheet	To preserve client dignity

Procedure	Rationale
Provided that the client can lie flat, remove all but one pillow and place remaining spare pillows to one side of the client's head	To facilitate easier moving, rolling
Gently roll client towards the nurse facing, taking care to maintain safety and supporting the head at all times. If the client is clinically obese it is advisable to raise the cot side. Check that any tubing/drips or drains are not being pulled and continually observe the client for any signs of undue distress	Safety and comfort of client
Change bottom sheet by rolling it to the centre of the bed	Reduces transmission of organisms
Lay clean sheet in the centre of the bed and, using centre-fold of the sheet as a guide, roll half the sheet to this centre-fold and tuck in the portion of sheet near side at top, bottom and side	Ease of securing
Ensure sheet flat, smooth, crease free	Prevent risk of pressure sores
Gently roll client towards the nurse on the opposite side of the bed, advising them of the 'bump' in the middle and remembering to support the client's head, and take the pillow with you	Safety and comfort of the client. To promote co-operation
Remove soiled sheet and place in linen skip immediately	Reduces risk of cross-infection
Unfold the remainder of the clean bottom sheet and fit to the bed, tucking in top and sides (as above) and ensuring that it remains smooth and crease free	Prevent risk of pressure sores
Roll client gently to the centre of the bed and replace soiled pillowcases whilst supporting the client's head	Client comfort and safety
Place clean top sheet over existing sheet and remove soiled top sheet	Client privacy
Make up as unoccupied bed, involving patient in choice of bedding, and avoiding tight bedding over lower limbs and feet	To meet individual needs of client. Enable movement of lower limbs and feet. Prevent pressure sores and possibility of plantar flexion
Lower bed to a suitable height for the client and ensure that the brake is on	Safety and access for client

Procedure	Rationale
Reposition the client to individual preference and in keeping with their medical condition and replace bed table, jug, magazines, tissues, etc. within client's reach, including call button	Client comfort and safety
Remove linen skip/equipment and leave area clean and tidy	Safety and ease of the client
Remove apron and wash hands	Prevent cross-infection

Disposal of linen

The correct disposal of linen plays an important part in infection control. Incorrect disposal of linen is a potential hazard, not only for clients but for all health care workers.

Equipment

Linen skip, appropriately coloured linen bags (check local policy), apron, plastic bag (for soiled linen), red alginate bag (soluble for infected linen), red linen bag (for infected linen) and gloves (if in contact with soiled or infected linen) are required. The procedures and rationales are given below.

Procedure	Rationale
Apply apron and wash hands	To reduce the risk of cross-infection and prevent contact with uniform
Take linen skip and appropriate linen bag to bedside	Linen can immediately be disposed of thus reducing the risk of cross-infection
If linen is soiled or infected don gloves	Reduces risk of contamination
When removing the linen always fold linen away from apron and place immediately in either a plastic bag for soiled linen or in red alginate bag/ soluble for infected linen (check local policy)	Reduces risk of contamination
Do not overfill bag and always seal alginate bags before leaving the bedside and do not mix clean, soiled and infected linen	Prevents potential leakage and reduces risk of cross-infection
Place in appropriate linen bag and remove to sluice area, seal when ¾ full and arrange removal by the portering staff	Reduces risk of contamination and reduces potential for back injury
Remove apron and wash hands	Reduces risk of cross-infection

Assisting individuals with bathing

Maintaining personal hygiene is essential for the preservation of health and the prevention of infection, and removal of body odour.

Individuals, whenever possible, should be encouraged to perform their own personal hygiene so that their independence is promoted. Bathing may involve assisted washes in or out of bed, bed bathing, showering or immersion in a general bath. Care must be taken throughout to keep wounds or dressings dry, and such considerations may influence the mode of choice.

Equipment

The equipment required will vary according to individual client needs but may include soap, face cloth, two towels (one face and one bath), disposable wipes, clinical waste disposable bags, toiletries (for example, deodorant, perfume, aftershave), client's comb/brush, bowl of hot water (35–40°C), gloves and apron, lotion thermometer, suitable bath/shower, chair/shower stool, disposable floor mat, appropriate aids if bathing/shaving, clean nightdress/pyjamas or clothing as required, clean bed linen/linen skip and a trolley/adequate surface. The procedures and rationales of bed bathing are given below.

Procedure	Rationale
Plan activity around client's daily routine and in line with other nursing activities	Promote normal routine and reduce unnecessary disturbance
Explain the procedure to the client	To gain informed consent and client's co-operation and participation in the activity
Collect and prepare the equipment	To ensure all equipment is ready to use
Prepare the environment so that it is warm. Close windows and ensure privacy	Avoids chilling the client
Adjust the height of the bed if necessary. Check brakes of bed are on	Client comfort and safety
Ensure adequate space around bed area for equipment	Easy, comfortable access
Ask client if they wish to empty their bladder and/or bowels and ensure that they are pain free before bathing	Client may otherwise be anxious and unco-operative during procedure
Help the client into a comfortable position	Client co-operation and easier access for the nurse

Procedure	Rationale
Remove bed linen but leave one sheet covering the client	To maintain client's privacy and dignity
Assist the client to remove nightwear if necessary	Client may be unable to do this without assistance
Be aware of intravenous lines, catheters, drains, injuries and client's level of mobility, and sequence removal of nightwear accordingly	To avoid injury and discontinuing lines
Fill the bowl and check the temperature of the water using lotion thermometer. If client is co-operative ask them if the water temperature is to their liking	Client comfort and safety. Meeting individual's preferences
Ask client if they use soap on their face before commencing	Negotiated care. Also, persistent use of some soaps can alter the pH of the skin leading to drying. Soap can also irritate the eyes
Involving the client as much as they desire and are able, wash the face, taking care to be particularly gentle around the eyes. Use a clean area of the cloth for each eye and clean the eyes from the inner to the outer canthus. Wash and check the ears. Rinse and dry	To promote independence and activity/ movement. Prevents debris being dragged into the tear ducts and pathogens being trans- ferred from one eye to the other. To prevent unnecessary cooling
Wash the neck. Rinse and dry	To prevent unnecessary cooling
Continue washing, rinsing and drying the client, exposing each area to be washed as follows:	Protects modesty and promotes dignity
Arms (wash from the hands, paying particu- lar attention to the nails), washing the arm furthest away from the nurse first;	Allows assistant to dry and reduces the risk of cooling
Chest and abdomen; continue in the same manner washing the back, lower limbs and feet, exposing only the area being washed	Ensures that all parts of the body are washed and moves from 'clean' to 'dirty' systematically, thus facilitating team working
A towel can be used to protect the bottom sheet during the procedure	This prevents the client having to lie on a wet sheet
Pay particular attention to the axillae, umbili- cus, skin folds of breasts, abdomen and groin, carefully rinsing flannel or disposing of wipes after each use	Axillae are usually heavily colonized by bacteria, therefore flannels should not be reused without cleansing. Wipes are better disposed of. Prevents odour, skin irritation. Prevents cross-infection

Procedure	Rationale
Change the water as it cools or becomes dirty	Prevents cooling of the client, increases cleanliness and promotes client comfort
Pay particular attention to the toenails and areas between the toes	To reduce the actual/potential pain and risk of infection. **NB** It is generally not acceptable to cut clients' nails due to risk of injury, particularly of those of clients with diabetes in whom wound healing is usually poor. Referral to a chiropodist is preferable (check local policy)
If desired and appropriate help client to immerse hands and feet in bowl of water, supporting the limbs	To promote relaxation and client comfort
Leave perineal hygiene until last. Change water, put on gloves and use disposable wipes. Always clean from front to back using as many wipes as necessary to cleanse the area	Prevents transmission of micro-organisms from anus to urethra
Dispose of soiled disposable materials including gloves into a clinical waste bag when finished	Prevention of cross-infection
Throughout procedure observe and assess the client's skin for blemishes, bruises, swelling and redness. If present report same and document in client's records	To monitor client's condition and reduce the likelihood of the development of pressure sores
Assist client to dress in clean nightwear/clothing of their choice. Apply deodorant/perfume/make-up in keeping with client preference	Promote patient comfort, independence and self-esteem
Change bed linen as necessary	Prevent cross-infection
Provide a mirror to encourage client to comb/brush hair in preferred style	Promotes self-esteem
If necessary assist client with brushing teeth and/or rinsing mouth (see 'Assisting individuals with oral hygiene', below)	To promote good oral hygiene
Remove all equipment and leave the area clean and tidy	Safety of the client and the environment. Prevents transmission of infection
Ensure that the client is comfortable with desired articles within easy reach	For ease of access and to promote client independence
Remove apron, wash hands	Prevent risk of cross-infection
Document client's reaction to the procedure in nursing care plan. Report any abnormal findings or adverse reactions and update care plan accordingly	Legal requirement. Facilitates good communication amongst health care staff

Bathing/showering in the bathroom

The client's preference may be for a general bath (sometimes referred to as an 'up bath' or shower. An assessment of the individual client's preference along with an assessment of their strength, mobility and mental capacity is essential prior to the carrying out of this activity. The nurse must ensure the client's safety at all times. The procedures and rationales of bathing/showering in the bathroom are given below.

Procedure	Rationale
Plan the activity with the client and explain the procedure	To gain consent and co-operation
Prepare a warm environment, and ensure that all equipment is in the bathroom/shower room prior to taking the client	Prevents cooling. Ensures privacy and client safety. Saves time and is therefore a more effective use of resources
Assist the client in gathering towels, clean clothing/nightwear and toiletries. Walk with the client to the bathing area (if appropriate). If the client has difficulty mobilizing, it may be necessary to use a mechanical hoist or wheelchair	Promotes independence and ensures client safety
Apply apron, wash hands and apply gloves as appropriate	Personal protection and prevention of cross-infection
Line the bath with a plastic liner and prepare the water for the bath/shower, monitoring the temperature using a lotion thermometer, and adjust to meet client's preferences.	Reduces potential for cross-infection. Promotes client safety and comfort
NB Always run cold water first and adjust to warm (approx. 30°C).	To prevent scalding
Assist client in undressing, but keep covered until immersed in water	To promote and maintain client independence and to maintain body temperature, client dignity and privacy
Assist client into bath or under the shower. Two nurses may be required for this activity (client may need to sit on hoist seat in the bath, or shower chair in the shower)	Client safety/comfort
Assist the client in washing, ensuring face, neck and upper body are washed first	To reduce risk of cross-contamination
If required, assist client in washing hair	To promote a sense of well-being and a positive body image

Procedure	Rationale
When finished, assist client out of bath/shower. Ensure towels are immediately available for drying	To promote client safety. To prevent body cooling
Assist client to dry as necessary paying particular attention to feet and in between toes	Leaving moist areas can lead to excoriation and infection
Encourage client to sit on chair, if unsteady, covered by a towel	Client safety, warmth and protection
Assist client to dress as desired	Promote independence, self-esteem
Assist the client in cleaning teeth/dentures either at sink, in bathroom or showering area (see below)	To promote good oral hygiene, client comfort and well-being
Assist the client in combing/brushing hair	To promote a positive self-image
Assist the client in gathering all toiletries before returning to client's bed area	Safety and security
Assist the client to chair or bed depending on client's preference and ensure they are left with their belongings within easy reach	Client comfort and safety
Remove any equipment from bathroom/shower area. Clean, dry or dispose of as required. Clean the bath out thoroughly	To reduce the risk of cross-infection
Remove apron and gloves and wash hands	Prevent risk of cross-infection
Record in nursing care records. Report any abnormal findings or adverse reactions	Legal requirement. Facilitates effective communication amongst health care staff

Assisted wash

Assessment of the client's abilities is crucial prior to facilitating them to independently undertake any aspect of their personal cleansing. This assessment must be undertaken by a health care professional who is knowledgeable about the person's medical condition, as the person may at first glance appear independent and indeed believe they are capable of self-care when they are at rest. However, for some clients, the slightest exertion can radically alter their ability to perform even the simplest task such as washing their face.

Assistance may be anything from merely providing them with the appropriate equipment and ensuring a safe environment, to washing the parts that they are unable to reach without causing undue distress, for example back, legs and hair.

Bathing a baby or child

In addition to the preservation of health and the prevention of infection, bath time for a small child offers an ideal opportunity for activities other than for their hygiene needs. The removal of drains, catheters, and dressings, or the passing of urine after surgery, are examples of activities that can be more easily undertaken during a bath. However, as with adults, care must be taken not to wet wounds or dressings that should be kept dry. Bath time is also an opportunity to play with and get to know the small or older child in a non-threatening environment. It also can have a calming effect on babies who are distressed by their unfamiliar environment.

The procedure for bathing a child is the same as for an adult but is usually undertaken with the use of bath toys. Toys that are used must be left to drain and thoroughly dried afterwards to prevent the growth of bacteria. The following procedure should be undertaken with newborn babies and babies up to the age of about six months. It can be modified to simply wash the baby's face and bottom, more commonly referred to as 'topping and tailing'.

Equipment

The equipment needed consists of mild baby soap or baby bath solution; clean towel; non-sterile eye swabs (not cotton wool); disposable wipes; clean nappy and disposal bag for the soiled one; change of clothing if required; container of sterile water; and a baby bath. The procedures and rationales of bathing/showering in the bathroom are given below.

Procedure	Rationale
Plan activities around the baby's daily routine and in line with other nursing activities	Promote normal routine and reduce unnecessary disturbance
Collect and prepare the equipment	Ensure all equipment is ready to use
Prepare the environment so that it is warm. Close windows	Avoids chilling the baby. Babies cannot shiver and they lose heat more quickly than an adult
Apply apron and wash hands. Apply gloves if required	Personal protection and prevention of cross-infection

Procedure	Rationale
Ensure that the baby bath is placed on a table or stand at a comfortable height when seated	Reduces the potential for back injury in the carer
Fill the baby bath with water that is comfortably warm. Test the temperature of the water with a bath thermometer or the elbow (approx. 30°C). Ensure that the hot and cold water is well mixed	Prevents scalding of the baby's skin
Ensure adequate space around the cot area for equipment	Easy comfortable access and accident prevention
Remove the baby's clothing and the nappy, placing it in a nappy disposal bag. Wipe away any faeces with a clean dry wipe if necessary. Always wipe the nappy area from front to back in girls	Faeces will contaminate the bath water if left on the skin. Faeces can enter the urethra causing urinary tract infection if wiping from back to front
Place the baby on the cot (or knees while seated) and wrap in a towel with the baby's arms inside the towel	Patient safety. Prevents heat loss
Throughout procedure observe/assess the baby's skin for blemishes, bruises, swelling and redness. If present report same and document in nursing records	To monitor baby's condition and reduce the likelihood of the development of pressure sores
Clean the eyes from the middle to the outer aspect using the swabs and sterile water. Do not use the same swab for both eyes	Prevents debris being dragged into the tear ducts and cross-infection occurring between each eye. Cotton wool should not be used as fibres can scratch the cornea
Wash the rest of the face and ears with a disposable wipe and water from the baby bath, taking care not to allow water to run into the mouth. Pat dry using the towel whilst paying particular attention to the skin folds	Water entering the mouth while reclined may cause the baby to choke. Leaving the skin folds wet can cause the skin to become sore
Hold the head over the bath and wet the scalp area. Use a baby shampoo if required and rinse well. The use of shampoo is not necessary with every bath. If the baby has 'cradle cap' medical advice must be sought	Over-use of shampoo can cause excessive drying of the skin. 'Cradle cap' is a skin condition caused by over-production of skin cells and requires specific treatment
Take the baby out of the towel and place in the baby bath by holding in the crook of the arm whilst holding his/her arm furthest away from you. Use your free arm to hold the baby by the ankles until in the bath	Provides support and prevents the baby from slipping into the bath. The ankles do not need holding in the bath and the hand is required to wash the baby

Procedure	Rationale
Wash the baby's body using the hand previously used to hold the baby's ankles. Soap is only required if the nappy area was soiled	If baby bath solution is used, the use of soap as well is unnecessary and may cause drying of the delicate skin
Remove the baby from the bath using the reverse of the above holding technique, taking extra care, as the baby is now very slippery	Patient safety and comfort
Place the baby on the towel and pat dry paying particular attention to the skin folds	Leaving the skin folds wet can cause the skin to become sore
Put on a clean nappy and dress the baby in clean clothes as quickly as possible	To prevent heat loss
Remove apron and wash hands	To reduce risk of cross-infection
Document baby's reactions to the procedure in nursing care plan and report any abnormal findings or adverse reactions. Update care plan as appropriate	Legal requirement. Facilitates good communication amongst health care staff

Assisting individuals with oral hygiene

Oral hygiene may involve the use of a toothbrush and paste, a mouth-wash or other mouth cleaning preparations, such as interdental sticks and floss, to achieve and maintain the cleanliness of the teeth or dentures, the gums, hard and soft palates and lips. It is considered an essential nursing procedure as an unkempt mouth can prove to be a serious health hazard over time for some individuals. Assessment and care of the oral cavity should therefore form part of a client's daily hygiene routine, and efficacy of interventions should be continuously evaluated.

The functions of the mouth are:

- breathing
- speaking
- eating
- tasting
- drinking
- smiling
- kissing.

A healthy mouth should:

- be pink and moist, including the tongue, oral mucosa and gums
- have teeth/dentures that are clean and free of debris
- have adequate salivation
- have lips that are smooth and moist
- display no evidence of difficulties with eating or swallowing.

In order to deliver appropriate oral hygiene, it is recommended that an oral assessment tool be used to identify a client's oral health status (see Figure 3.1). The following are some of the specific points to consider when assessing an individual's oral hygiene:

- *Physical*
  fluid and dietary intake
  medication – some drugs can alter oral hygiene needs, including antibiotics,
    steroids, diuretics, drugs used in cytotoxic therapy, antihistamines, anti-
    spasmodics, anticholinergics, psychotropics, antidepressants,
    tranquillizers and opiates
  client receiving oxygen therapy or oral suction
  level of consciousness
  immune status
  physical disabilities, for example unable to move tongue from side to side,
    unable to empty oral cavity when eating
  health status; note particularly any renal impairment, diabetes or anaemia
  does the client have a tracheostomy?
  have they had a laryngectomy?
  ability to self-care
  surgery – oral, upper gastro-intestinal
  manual dexterity
  smoking
  age
  dentures/braces, full/partial, well fitting/ill fitting
  condition of lips, mucous membranes, gums, hard and soft palates
    (smooth/pink/moist/dry/cracked/ulcerated/bleeding)

- *Psychological*
  confusion
  disorientation
  depression
  level of self-esteem
  perceptions of self

- *Sociocultural*
  health benefits
  values
  dietary beliefs

Figure 3.1 Example of an oral assessment tool

Score	4	3	2	1
Patient's age	16-29	30-49	50-69	70+
Normal oral status	Good	Fair	Poor	Very poor
Ability to masticate	Full	Slightly limited	Very limited	Immobile
Nutritional status including hydration	Good	Fair	Poor	Very poor
Airway	Normal	Receiving humidified oxygen	Endotracheal tube in situ	Open mouth breathing

Subtotal

Does the client have:

      Anaemia?

      Immunosuppression?

      Diabetes?

      Renal impairment?

      Epilepsy?

Are they receiving any medication that might compromise their oral hygiene status, for example antibiotics, steroids?

Subtract 1 from the subtotal for each point noted

Client's total 'at risk' score

Score: 15 or above – provide/encourage three-hourly mouth care; 12-14 – provide/encourage two-hourly mouth care; below 12 – provide/encourage hourly mouth care

- *Environmental*
  availability of clean/running water supply
  other resources, for example toothbrushes, toothpaste
  privacy
- *Politico-economic*
  limited finances for a healthy diet or resources

Performing oral hygiene

Performing oral hygiene can help to maintain healthy structures of the oral cavity, retain moisture, remove debris, prevent plaque and reduce the risk of infection, as well as adding to the client's comfort and well-being. Clients should be encouraged to perform oral hygiene immediately after eating and more frequently if their health is compromised. Toothpaste, toothbrush and water are the cheapest, most reliable and most effective tools for mouth care, though a doctor, dentist or dental hygienist may sometimes recommend other products from time to time if a client's oral hygiene is compromised (see Table 3.1). National standards for oral hygiene, and for personal hygiene, have been developed by the Department of Health. These can be accessed at www.doh.gov.uk/essenceofcare.

The equipment needed consists of spatula/torch for oral inspection; disposable gloves and apron; solutions/cleaning agents/mouthwash (all solutions should be freshly prepared in accordance with manufacturers' instructions); toothpaste, denture cleaners; paper towels; clinical waste bag; water (drinking); denture pot if required – labelled; Vaseline/soft white paraffin gel; towel or protective clothing; tissues for wiping the mouth; suction equipment (if needed); airway (if needed); and an oral toilet pack if needed (this may already contain paper towels, disposal bag). The procedures and rationales for performing oral hygiene are given below.

Procedure	Rationale
Offer a full explanation of the procedure, including client's individual preferences	To gain consent, co-operation and participation in care
Ensure all equipment is at hand to administer care	To ensure effective use of time and resources
Apply apron, wash your hands and put on gloves	To prevent contamination with body fluids
Ensure privacy	To promote client dignity and self-esteem
Assist the client into a comfortable sitting position if possible	To promote client comfort and safety and to facilitate thorough oral inspection and assessment
Remove all appliances, e.g. dentures, and place in a labelled pot	To assist assessment of condition of the oral cavity
Using spatula and torch inspect oral cavity, including teeth, gums and mucosa. Note bleeding, ulcers, sores, food debris, condition of lips	Comprehensive assessment is essential to determine individual care needs

Procedure	Rationale
Place towel over client's chest	To protect clothing
Using a soft toothbrush and fluoride toothpaste gently brush all teeth at an angle of 45° to the teeth and all other surfaces, i.e. gums, tongue, and oral tissues. **NB** When cleaning the tongue, avoid the posterior aspect as this can stimulate the gag reflex	Effective in dislodging debris and dental plaque from teeth and the gingival margin. Encourages tissue perfusion. Client comfort
If the client cannot tolerate a toothbrush a foam stick can be used, though these are less effective	Client safety. To prevent inhalation of fluid
Offer the client water or mouthwash and advise them not to swallow this. Provide a receiver for disposal. Protect the airway at all times. Suction equipment may be used to remove any excess	Reduce potential for infection. Client safety. To prevent inhalation of fluid
Provide wipes or tissues and assist client to wash/wipe and dry mouth	Client comfort and dignity
Apply lubricant to lips	Helps moisturize the lips and can reduce potential for cracking
Toothbrushes should be rinsed and dried after use	Prevents growth of micro-organisms
Tidy area and clear away equipment	Safety
Remove gloves, apron and wash hands	Prevents cross-infection
Record procedure, listing any improvement or deterioration in the condition of the client's mouth	Legal requirement. Facilitates effective communication between health care staff

The frequency of this procedure should be based on regular oral cavity assessment and client preferences. In order to maintain a moist and healthy oral cavity clients should be encouraged to take frequent sips of fluids. Alternatively, soda water or ice cubes can be offered to freshen the mouth. Sucking on fresh fruit, if allowed, can also provide refreshment and helps stimulate saliva production, particularly pineapple.

Mouthwashes

A variety of mouthwash solutions are available on the market (see Table 3.1). Selection of mouthwash should be based on the following factors:

1 a thorough oral assessment
2 nurses' knowledge base regarding the suitability of a particular solution for a client
3 clients' preferences
4 individual prescription.

Table 3.1 Preparations for maintaining oral hygiene

Preparation	Uses	Disadvantages
Sodium bicarbonate	Effective mucosolvent	Tastes unpleasant and can burn if not adequately diluted. Can also alter oral pH allowing bacteria to multiply
Glycerine and thymol	Initially refreshing but effect lasts only 20-30 seconds	Can over-stimulate the salivary glands leading to reflex action and exhaustion
Tap water	Refreshing, ideal pH and readily available	Short lasting and does not contain a bactericide
Chlorhexidine gluconate	Inhibits bacterial growth	Tastes unpleasant and stains teeth with prolonged use
Synthetic saliva	Provides moisture	Does not check bacterial growth
Pineapple cubes/juice	Refreshing, promotes saliva production and contains an enzyme that helps cleanse the mouth	Cannot be used for clients who are nil by mouth
Petroleum jelly/Lip balm	Can prevent cracked lips	Some clients do not like the feel or taste
Toothpaste	Effective for removing debris	Can dry the oral cavity if not adequately rinsed
Nystatin	Effective for fungal infections	Tastes unpleasant to some clients. Must be prescribed
Denture cleaner/ Baking soda	Effective in removing stains	Can bleach dentures over time

It is important that the mouthwash solution is constituted according to the manufacturer's instructions and its use is monitored and evaluated. Some solutions, such as chlorhexidine gluconate, are classed as medications and should therefore always be prescribed and administered in accordance with local drug administration policies.

In promoting cleanliness and comfort, clients may use or be encouraged to use other mouth care aids such as dental floss. Flossing helps remove plaque and tartar between the teeth and thus reduces the potential for gum inflammation and infection. Flossing can be performed prior to or following teeth cleansing. The procedures and rationales for flossing are given below.

Procedure	Rationale
Discuss with client their preferred technique	To gain co-operation and consent and to facilitate negotiation
Put on apron and wash hands. Wear gloves if performing procedure for client	Reduces risk of cross-infection. Reduces transmission of organisms
Remove a length of dental floss, wrap around both index fingers (either client or nurse), insert one end between teeth and gently slide up and down each side of every tooth	Avoids injury to the gums
Adjust floss between index fingers	To facilitate control
Continue until all teeth have been flossed. A fresh part of floss is used for each tooth	To reduce potential for cross-infection
Allow client to rinse after flossing	To remove residual debris and promote client comfort
Provide facilities for the client to wash their hands following the procedure	Infection control
Note condition of teeth and gums and refer as appropriate	To ensure care needs are met

Care of dentures

An important aspect of oral hygiene is the care of prostheses, which include dentures, plates and braces. These are the client's personal property and need to be handled carefully to avoid damage and breakage. The procedures and rationales for denture care are given below.

Procedure	Rationale
Having washed hands and donned gloves, ask the client to remove prostheses and assist if necessary	Infection control
NB Some clients may be embarrassed about removing these in the presence of others; if this is the case ensure privacy	To promote dignity and maintain self-image
Always clean dentures in or over a plastic or disposable receptacle	Once wet they become very slippery and can easily be damaged if cleaned in or over a sink
Can be cleaned with a non-scented soap and water using a soft toothbrush, then rinsed well with fresh water	Non-irritant
When not in use, dentures/plates should be stored in cold water in a suitable labelled container. Do not allow dentures to dry out. A denture-soaking solution may be used but prostheses should not be left soaking in this for longer than the manufacturer's recommendation. Thorough rinsing is required before replacing in the mouth	To prevent shrinkage/warping and bacterial build-up. Gives gums a rest. Over-use of such solutions can cause discoloration and deterioration. Facilitates easier insertion
Clean gums, tongue and oral mucosa using a soft toothbrush and water as discussed above	To prevent re-introduction of infection and to stimulate blood flow to the gums
Always encourage clients to remove dentures/plate at night	To facilitate rest of the tissues and allow oxygenation of the hard/soft palates

Note that mouth care on unconscious clients should be undertaken with great caution and preferably in the presence of a registered practitioner. Suction equipment should always be at hand as there can be a significant risk of aspiration or choking in this client group.

Assisting individuals with eye care

Eye care is part of maintaining a client's personal hygiene and is usually performed as part of bathing/showering. Generally the normal physiological processes of blinking and tear production maintain the cleanliness of the eyes, along with daily washing. When a client has difficulty in meeting their eye care needs then the nurse may need to assist, particularly if discharges or crusts appear around the eyes. This can usually be removed by gentle eye swabbing, as outlined below.

The client's ability to see, along with any aids that are used by the client, such as glasses, contact lenses or eye glass, should be considered when assessing an individual's personal cleansing and dressing needs, and advice should be sought regarding the appropriate methods of cleaning these if unsure.

Removal of contact lenses is a skilled task; if uncertain as to how to proceed it is best to ask the client, relative (if knowledgeable) or other member of the health care team to demonstrate rather than risking damaging the conjunctiva or cornea.

Equipment

The equipment needed consists of sterile eye-dressing packs, sterile 0.9 per cent sodium chloride, tray for equipment, clinical waste bag and gloves (if risk of contact with blood or body fluids). The procedures and rationales for eye care are given below.

Procedure	Rationale
Explain procedure to client	To gain consent and co-operation
Apply apron and wash hands	To reduce risk of cross-infection
Gather all equipment	Ease of access
Ensure privacy for the client	Maintains dignity
Ensure good light source	To facilitate the procedure
Assist the client into a comfortable position	Client comfort, co-operation and ease of access for the nurse to perform the procedure
Prepare equipment, wash hands	To prevent cross-infection
Cover the client's chest using the towel from dressing pack	To protect client's clothing
Instruct client to close their eyes	To reduce the risk of damaging the conjunctiva or cornea
Moisten swab in the solution and gently swab from the inner canthus outwards, using one wipe. Repeat in the same direction until the eye is free from crusts/discharge. Repeat on the other eye, all the time observing the general condition of the eyes	To restore hygiene

Procedure	Rationale
If the client has an infection, wash hands before moving from one eye to the other and always swab the non-infected eye first	To decrease the risk of infecting the other eye
If the eye is to be touched to remove a foreign body, a cotton bud should be used	To prevent further injury or abrasion
Gently dry the client's eyelids	To remove any excess moisture
Remove and dispose of equipment safely	Infection control
Leave the client comfortable. Remove apron and wash hands	To reduce the risk of cross-infection
Evaluate care delivery, document and report any change in client's condition	Legal requirement
Update care plan as necessary	Promotes continuity of care

If unsure of the client's care needs or unsure of the procedure it is imperative that a specialist be consulted.

Facial shaving

Facial shaving is often a significant aspect of a man's personal hygiene routine and can improve both his comfort and self-esteem. It can be performed during or following washing. In assessing a client's needs the following should be considered:

1 The frequency of shaving. Clients without beards usually shave daily but clients with moustaches and beards should not be ignored, as they also require daily grooming. It is important to assess the religious and cultural beliefs of clients in relation to the management of body hair to avoid causing offence.

2 The client's ability to manipulate a razor.

3 The client's safety in handling equipment and performing facial shaving, for example an electric razor may be preferable if the client is unstable.

4 The condition of the client's skin, for example raised areas, pimples, rashes.

5 Wet shaving is not recommended for clients with a bleeding disorder, epilepsy or neuromuscular disorder such as Parkinson's disease as the risk of injury is significantly increased.

Some medications and disorders can induce the growth of facial hair in women. This clearly needs addressing tactfully and diplomatically.

The equipment usually consists of apron, mirror, electric razor with clean cutting heads (preferably client's own) and/or disposable razor, towel for protection, shaving cream or soap (if wet shaving), aftershave lotion, skin conditioner (if desired), bowl and wipes/face flannel. The procedures and rationales for facial shaving are given below. To reduce the likelihood of injury these procedures should only be undertaken by a skilled person.

Procedure	Rationale
Explain the procedure to the client	To gain consent and co-operation
Wash hands	Infection control
Put on apron	Nurse protection
Assist client in assembling equipment, allowing for individual preferences and nuances	Client control and independence
Assist the client into a sitting position, and provide privacy	Ensures easy access and promotes dignity
Protect client's upper chest and shoulders with towel	Reduces laundering
Ensure good lighting	Promotes safety
Encourage client to shave himself if possible	Promotes independence
Client's own equipment should be used. Communal razors and shaving brushes should not be used	Reduces risk of cross-infection
If the nurse is performing the shave ask the client about individual preferences, e.g. which area of the face he shaves first	Promotes client involvement in decision-making and ensures individual's needs are met
Prepare warm water in bowl (approx. 30ºC). Assist/encourage client to wash face with warm water and wipes/face flannel	Warm cloth helps soften the skin and prevents pulling
If assisting apply shaving cream and/or soap ensuring a good lather over face, chin, under nose, neck	Encourages the hairs to stand on end for ease of removal and reduces skin irritation

Procedure	Rationale
Hold razor in dominant hand and at a 45° angle to the skin, use short, firm strokes in the direction of hair growth, keeping the skin taut with the other hand (if client has tendency to bleed, nurse should wear disposable gloves or better still discourage wet shaving)	Prevents razor cuts and discomfort during shaving
Allow client to look in the mirror to monitor progress. While performing shave suggest that the client raise a hand if it becomes uncomfortable at any time or if they wish to cough	Promotes client participation and involvement. To prevent injury
Rinse razor in bowl of warm water at frequent intervals. The nurse may need to change the razor and/or apply more lather	Maintains a clean-cutting razor blade
Repeat the above until all facial hair is removed and the client is satisfied. Rinse the face thoroughly, ensuring all soap and hair has been removed	Prevents accumulation of shaving cream, which can cause drying
Gently pat the skin dry using the face towel	Moisture may cause sore skin
Apply aftershave lotion/skin conditioner if required. Allow client to look in mirror to see if they are satisfied with their personal appearance	Stimulates/lubricates the skin. Promotes self-image/esteem
Remove all equipment. Leave client comfortable and the environment dry. Return client's toiletries. Discard disposable razor in sharps box	Safety
Remove gloves and apron, and wash hands	To prevent cross-infection
Record in nursing records as part of maintaining personal hygiene and report any anomalies	Legal requirement

Note that if the client is using an electric shaver, the skin should be kept dry and the shaver should be cleaned immediately following use.

Hair care

Hair care is again a significant part of the grooming process and the attention given to this activity often reflects how a client feels. The condition of the hair and scalp can also be a good indicator of a client's general health; therefore regular attention to this aspect of care is important.

The client's gender, cultural and racial preferences need to be taken into account when assisting in grooming of the hair, and under no circumstances should a client's hair be cut without their express permission. The client's level of independence needs to be considered when undertaking your initial and subsequent assessments, along with any contra-indications to this procedure, such as arthritis or head and neck injuries, which may affect their ability to become involved.

Washing the client's hair may take place whilst they are confined to bed or, if mobile, the client can be accompanied to the washroom and sit at the sink.

Equipment

In order to wash a client's hair in bed, the following equipment is needed:

- face flannel
- towels
- shampoo/hair conditioner
- bowl of warm water for pouring
- container or inflatable shampooette to collect used water
- jug of water
- waterproof sheeting to protect bed
- plastic apron
- brush/comb
- surface for equipment
- hairdryer.

Two nurses can best perform this procedure, as one can support the client's head whilst the other pours the water, shampoo, etc. The procedures and rationales for washing hair are given below.

Procedure	Rationale
Explain procedure to the client	Gain consent and co-operation
Gather all the equipment at the bedside	Ease of access, ready for use
Put on apron, wash hands. Ensure client's privacy	Reduce risk of cross-infection

Procedure	Rationale
Adjust the height of the bed, remove bed head and assist the client into a supported, comfortable position with their head protruding over the top edge of bed	Ease of procedure
Place waterproof sheeting under client's shoulders, neck and head	Protection of pillows, bedclothes and client's clothing
Place towel over client's chest, up to the chin and around the shoulders. You may need to place a rolled towel underneath the client's neck for support	Support and comfort
Place bowl or shampooette under the client's head	To catch water as it is poured over the client's head
Inspect the client's hair and scalp, removing any hair accessories	To assess the necessity for special shampoos/treatments. Ease of access. To prevent trauma
Brush and/or comb client's hair through	To remove tangles and allow shampoo to permeate through the hair
Talk client through each step of the procedure. Assess the temperature of the water with the client. Ask client to hold face flannel over the eyes as water is poured over the client's head. Completely wet head and then apply shampoo, lather well. Monitor client's condition throughout the procedure and stop if any sign of undue distress	Client co-operation, client safety. Prevent water and shampoo irritating the eyes. To maintain comfort
Massage scalp by applying fingertip pressure all over the head. Rinse thoroughly and repeat. Apply hair conditioner if desired	To ensure thorough distribution of shampoo
Rinse hair thoroughly and dry face using clean tissues	Residual shampoo can dry the scalp and increase the potential for dandruff
Towel the hair dry	To prevent cooling
Assist the client into a comfortable position and comb hair through	Client comfort. Removal of tangles
Dry the hair using a hairdryer and/or assist to style in client's preferred style; show in mirror	Promote client choice. Maintain body image and self-esteem

Procedure	Rationale
Remove all equipment, leaving area clean and dry	Maintain a safe environment
Remove apron and wash hands	To prevent cross-infection
Evaluate care delivery and document in nursing care records	Legal requirement and promotion of continuity of care

Infestation with head lice can be successfully treated with proprietary medications such as Benzyl Benzoate, Malathion, Carbaryl or Permethrin.

Assisting individuals to dress

Dressing allows the client to maintain their individuality, self-image and self-esteem besides providing protection. It is an important vehicle for communicating one's personality, values, beliefs and culture in society, as well as one's gender. Nurses can assist clients in this activity by encouraging them to make choices and decisions about their personal dress and assisting them in this activity when they are unable to self-care.

Dressing best takes place following washing or bathing though clothes should always be changed when soiled, to promote the client's dignity. Clothes worn during waking hours should not be worn for sleeping as one can lose up to one litre of sweat during the night and this can increase significantly in illness.

When dressing the client in clothing of their choosing bear in mind that the clothes should be in keeping with the environment, the general condition of the client and the time of day. Also consider their ease of removal and application and the need for access, for example intravenous cannulation, catheters and drains. The procedures and rationales for assisting clients to dress are given below.

Procedure	Rationale
Assist the client to select suitable clothes. This may be their own personal clothing or clothing from the clinical area's supplies. **NB** If personal clothing is used great care should be taken to ensure that this does not find its way into the general laundering system	To include them in active decision-making and promote individuality

Procedure	Rationale
Ensure privacy	Dignity of client
Assist client to remove soiled clothing, outer garments first. If necessary assist in cleansing prior to redressing	To maintain hygiene
Have clothing available and ready to use. If client has limited mobility or limb injuries as identified during their mobility assessment (see Chapter 2), remove clothing from unaffected side first	Prevents unnecessary cooling of the client. Avoids injury
Be aware of wounds, drains and indwelling catheters when removing clothing and re-dressing client	To avoid discomfort and disturbance
Give the client time, and encourage them to perform as much of the activity as possible	To promote independence and self-care
Remove clothing in a systematic way, e.g. top to bottom, replacing with clean clothing as each item is removed. If personal clothing is removed ensure these are stored safely in client's locker prior to laundering	Prevents unnecessary cooling
Choose clothing with easy fitting fastenings, e.g. Velcro fasteners, rather than buttons and/or loose sleeves if appropriate (if client has difficulty with traditional fastenings)	To promote independence and self-care
Give client access to mirror to check overall appearance	Confirm approval. Promote positive self-image
Ensure client is left comfortable. Record any changed care needs in nursing record	To ensure continuity of care

References and further reading

Adams R (1996) Qualified nurses lack adequate knowledge related to oral hygiene, resulting in inadequate oral care of patients on medical wards. Journal of Advanced Nursing 24: 552-60.

Allen K (1993) Oral health for people with learning disabilities. In Hallas D (1993) Caring for People with Mental Handicaps. London: Butterworth.

British Society for Disability and Oral Health (2000a) Guidelines for Oral Health for Long-stay Patients and Residents, revised edn. London: British Society for Disability and Oral Health.

British Society for Disability and Oral Health (2000b) Guidelines for the Development of Standards for Oral Health Care for Dependent, Dysphagic, Critically and Terminally Ill Patients, revised edn. London: British Society for Disability and Oral Health.

British Society for Disability and Oral Health (2000c) The Development of Standards for Domiciliary Dental Care Services: Guidelines and Recommendations, revised edn. London: British Society for Disability and Oral Health.

British Society for Disability and Oral Health (2000d) Oral Health Care for People with Mental Health Problems: Guidelines and Recommendations, revised edn. London: British Society for Disability and Oral Health.

British Society for Disability and Oral Health (2000e) Oral Health Care for People with a Physical Disability: Guidelines and Recommendations, revised edn. London: British Society for Disability and Oral Health.

Campbell S, Glasper E (Eds) (1995) Whaley and Wong's Children's Nursing. London: Mosby.

Department of Health (2001) Essence of Care. Patient focused benchmarking for health care practitioners. http://www.doh.gov.uk/essenceofcare.

Elkin M, Perry A, Potter P (2000) Nursing Interventions and Clinical Skills, 2nd edn. St Louis, IL: Mosby.

Evans G (2001) A rationale for oral care. Nursing Standard 15(43): 33-6.

Field D (1998) Mouth care. Nursing Times 94(2): 18-24.

Huband S, Trigg E (eds) (2000) Practices in Children's Nursing: Guidelines for Hospital and Community Nurses. Edinburgh: Churchill Livingstone.

Jamieson E, McCall JM, Whyte LA (2002) Clinical Nursing Practices, 4th edn. Edinburgh: Churchill Livingstone.

Jevon P, Jevon M (2001) Facial shaving. Nursing Times 97(11): 43-4.

Jones C (1998) The importance of oral hygiene in nutritional support. British Journal of Nursing 7(2): 74-83.

Mallet J, Dougherty L (2000) The Royal Marsden Hospital Manual of Clinical Nursing Procedures, 5th edn. Oxford: Blackwell Science.

Millar B (2000) Coming clean. Nursing Times 96: 24-6.

Moules T, Ramsay J (1998) The Textbook of Children's Nursing. Cheltenham: Stanley Thornes.

Pearson LS (1996) A comparison of the ability of foam swabs and toothbrushes to remove dental plaque: implications for nursing practice. Journal of Advanced Nursing 23: 62-9.

Perry A, Potter P (2002) Clinical Nursing Skills and Techniques, 5th edn. St Louis, IL: Mosby.

Shaw K (1999) Oral Hygiene: Principles for Effective Practice. Rotherham: Rotherham General Hospitals NHS Trust.

Whiting L (1999) Maintaining patients' personal hygiene. Professional Nurse 14(5): 338-40.

WHO (World Health Organization) (1988) Oral Health - Global Indicators for Health. Geneva: WHO.

Wolf ZR (1997) Nursing students experience bathing patients for the first time. Nurse Educator 22(2): 41-6.

Chapter 4

Maintaining a safe environment

Julie Foster and Penelope Ann Hilton

Introduction

The skills required for maintaining a safe environment cover a wide range of activities. Some of the activities within this chapter explain how to examine and monitor a client's condition, thus maintaining their personal safety and well-being, whilst others are concerned with maintaining the safety and well-being of self, colleagues and visitors as well as of clients. These activities generally fall into one of two categories: those issues that are related to the internal environment, for example blood pressure monitoring, and those concerned with the external environment, for example fire. The reader is reminded to consult the Department of Health's six benchmarks for best practice (see http://www.doh.gov.uk/essenceofcare) when caring for clients with mental health needs.

The impact and applicability of some of the points in this chapter as they relate to health care, particularly some of those underpinned by government legislation and policy, may seem less obvious at first glance. Nevertheless, by examining such issues we can soon identify how health care professionals are involved in the maintenance of a safe environment on a daily basis in keeping with such legislation.

By the end of this chapter, it is hoped that your knowledge and understanding of the role in maintaining a safe environment of care will have been increased; a greater awareness of responsibilities towards clients, their families, their friends, and colleagues working alongside you will have been developed; and that there will be a greater awareness of the skills necessary to minimize the potential for such incidents. Unfortunately, despite best intentions, occasionally untoward incidents do occur. Provided the correct procedures and evidence-based practices have been followed as outlined here and in your local policy manual, and that the procedure for reporting such occurrences is followed, then there should be nothing to fear.

The factors that may affect maintenance of a safe environment may be:

- *Physical,* arising from alteration in the structure, function or processes of the bodily systems
- *Psychological,* such as anxiety or aggression
- *Sociocultural,* for example family support, health, beliefs
- *Environmental,* including smoking, spillages and safety during investigative procedures
- *Politico-economic,* for example lack of finances, social support, government policies.

The chapter commences by giving some of the common terminology associated with the activity of maintaining a safe environment, before addressing issues surrounding personal safety and the basic principles of health and safety at work. It then deals with issues surrounding infection control; monitoring of clients' pulses and blood pressures; how to respond in the event of a cardiopulmonary arrest; issues surrounding the safe storage of medicines; how to respond in the event of a fire; and, finally, assessing an individual's ability to maintain a safe environment. The chapter concludes with references and suggestions for further reading.

Common terminology

Amniotic fluid	A bodily fluid which surrounds the foetus during pregnancy
Asepsis	Freedom from disease-causing organisms
Cardiopulmonary	Related to the heart and lungs
Cerebrospinal fluid	A bodily fluid found in the spinal column and brain
Cytotoxic	Chemicals which destroy cells
Endogenous	From within
Exogenous	From an external source
Nosocomial infection	Hospital-acquired infection
Paracentesis	Procedure involving the puncturing of a cavity wall to drain or remove bodily fluid
Peritoneal fluid	A bodily fluid found within the perineum in some disorders
Sepsis	Infection
Synovial fluid	A bodily fluid found in a joint, e.g. knee
Universal precautions	Locally, nationally and internationally acknowledged guidelines aimed at reducing the risk of cross-infection, contamination or injury within health care settings

Personal safety

For many people, embarking on a career in health care involves moving to a new location be it a new town, city or home, or it may simply involve travelling to new areas at different times of day or night. Though often neglected in the exciting milieu, consideration of personal safety should be paramount if we are to be of any help to others. The following section offers some simple precautions that one can take to maximize personal safety and which can be shared with others.

Thinking about such possible dangers can sometimes provoke fear and anxiety even in the most confident individuals. It is therefore important to remind the reader at this juncture to keep things in perspective.

1 **Get to know the area**
   - Walk with a friend and become familiar with the local area, including the whereabouts of telephones in case of an emergency.
   - Know secluded areas to avoid, and walk in well-lit areas.
   - Talk with a friend about strategies you might use in various situations. Are there any escape routes you could use if forced into a corner?
   - A map of the area you plan on visiting can be helpful in planning for an emergency.

2 **Planning and preparation**
   - Let someone know where you are going and when you will be back. If possible give a contact number.
   - If you wear a personal stereo, remember you can't hear traffic, or somebody approaching behind you. You can therefore easily be surprised.
   - If you want to wear jewellery, conceal it until you reach your destination.
   - If you often walk home in the dark, get a personal attack alarm. Carry it in your hand so you can use it immediately to scare off an attacker. Make sure it is designed to continue sounding if it's dropped or falls to the ground, and, most importantly, that you know how to use it.
   - Before you leave home, remove things from your bag or holdall that you won't need that day. The less you carry, the less you have to lose and the less hesitant you will be if you have to give up your bag or wallet.
   - Always keep at least one arm free. Do not load yourself with packages.
   - Backpacks with back pockets are easy targets for thieves, especially in crowded subways or buses. Take the pack off when stationary or in a group of people.
   - Choose a bag with a flap and secure fastener. Carry your bag toward the front of your body with the clasp facing inwards, not bouncing against your back.

- Carry your house keys in your pocket and don't carry house keys and means of your identity together. Put your chequebook, credit cards and correspondence into a separate pocket.
- Make sure your mobile is fully charged if you have one.

3 **Posture and attitude**
- Attackers will target vulnerable people. Act confident even if you are scared.
- Walk assertively, head up and shoulders back. Stay aware, scan your path and stay in the middle of the path away from shrubs and bushes, etc.
- Set your face; make it appear serious and strong.
- Make eye contact and do not look down. Looking down shows you are intimidated.
- Develop your own strong, confident look and practise this in the mirror.
- Make brief eye contact as you walk. Make sure they know that you know they are there.

4 **When you are out and about**
- If you regularly go jogging or cycling try to vary your route and time. Stick to well-lit roads with pavements. On commons and parklands, keep to main paths and open spaces where you can see and be seen by other people – avoid wooded areas.
- Do not take short cuts through dark alleys, parks or across waste ground.
- Walk facing the traffic so a car cannot pull up behind you unnoticed.
- Do not hitchhike or take lifts from strangers.
- If someone grabs your bag, let it go. Remember your safety is more important than your property.
- If you think someone is following you, check by crossing the street, more than once if necessary, to see if he or she follows you. If you are still worried, get to the nearest place where there are other people, a pub or anywhere with a lot of lights on, and call the police.
- If a car stops and you are threatened, scream and shout, and set off your personal attack alarm if you have one. Get away as quickly as you can. This will gain you vital seconds and make it more difficult for the car driver to follow. If you can, make a mental note of the number and description of the car. Write down details as soon as possible afterwards.

5 **Going to your car**
- Approach the car with your keys in your hand.
- Scan the area around the car as you get closer and glance under the car to see that no one is hiding.
- Be aware of people approaching you, and asking for directions.
- In general be aware of anyone getting too close to you as you get into your car. Keep at least two-arms' length distance away from them.
- Check the interior of the car before opening the door. Make this a habit.

- Always load your packages in the car before you put children inside. If your car gets carjacked, at least your family will be safe.
- While driving, particularly in slow traffic or when stopped at traffic lights or junctions, keep your doors locked and the windows at least partway up.

6 **When driving**
- Before a long trip, make sure your vehicle is in good condition.
- Plan how to get to your destination before leaving, and stay on main roads if you can.
- Make sure you have enough money and petrol. Carry a spare petrol can.
- Keep change and a phone card in case you need to make a phone call.
- Carry a torch.
- Before you leave, tell anyone you are planning to meet what time you think you will get there and the route you are taking.
- If someone tries to flag you down, drive on until you come to a service station, or somewhere busy, and call the police. Do not pick up hitchhikers.
- Keep doors locked when driving and keep any bag or valuables out of sight. If you have the window open, only wind it down a little. Do not wind it down far enough to allow someone to reach in while you are stopped in traffic.
- If you think you are being followed, try to alert others by flashing your lights and sounding your horn. Make as much noise as possible. If you can, keep driving until you come to a busy place, or head for your nearest police, fire or ambulance station.
- After dark, park in a well-lit, busy place. Look around before you get out. If you are parking in daylight, but coming back for your car at night, think about how things will look in the dark.
- Have your key ready when you go back to your car. Check there is no one in the car.
- If the car develops problems, find a telephone. On motorways follow the marker arrows to the closest phone. They are never placed any more than a mile apart, on opposite sides of the motorway. Never cross the carriage-way to use a phone.
- While on the hard shoulder or telephoning, keep a sharp lookout and do not accept lifts from strangers. Wait for the police or breakdown service. Do not wait in the car, as there is a high risk of an accident. Wait on the embankment nearby with the front passenger door open.
- If someone approaches you or you feel threatened, return to your car, lock yourself in and speak to him or her through a small gap in the window.
- If you frequently have to travel after dark, consider carrying a mobile phone.

7 **Staying safe in taxis**
- If you are going to be out late, try to arrange a lift home or book a taxi.

Check that the taxi that arrives is the one you ordered. It is worthwhile asking for a description of the car, the colour, make, etc. and check this when it arrives.

- If you gave your name when you booked, check that the driver can tell you it before you get in.
- Always sit behind the driver. If you feel uneasy, ask to be let out in a well-lit area where there are plenty of people.
- If in doubt, do not get in the taxi.
- When you get home, ask the driver to wait until you are inside.
- There are a small number of disreputable mini-cab or private hire cars that tout for business; try to avoid them if at all possible.
- Always trust your instincts.

8 **Staying safe on public transport**
- Try to stay away from isolated bus stops, especially after dark.
- Do not sit alone. On buses, sit behind the driver or with friends. Do not fall asleep.
- As you arrive at your destination, scan the stop for anyone lurking. If you spot someone suspicious or feel apprehensive, stay on board or ask the driver to wait a few moments before pulling away.
- On an empty bus, sit near the driver or conductor.
- On a train, sit in a compartment where there are several other people – ideally one that will be near the exit of your destination. Check to see where the emergency lever or chain is situated.

9 **Using cash machines (ATMs)**
- Whenever possible, use well-lit, busy automated teller machines (ATMs) in well-populated locations during daylight hours. Avoid ATMs that are surrounded by shrubbery or trees, and do not use ATMs at the rear entrances of buildings or banks.
- Be aware of your surroundings and look around frequently.
- Use your body to block the screen when entering your code.
- Put your money away immediately.
- Do not count your money at the machine or sit in a parked car near an ATM.

10 **Staying safe at home**
- Make sure your house or flat is secure. Always secure outside doors. Fit barrel locks top and bottom. If you have to use a key, keep it nearby: you may need to get out quickly in the event of fire.
- If other people such as previous tenants could still have keys that fit, change the locks.
- Do not give keys to workmen or tradesmen, as they can easily make copies.
- If you wake to hear the sound of an intruder, only you can decide how

best to handle the situation. You may want to lie quietly to avoid attracting attention to yourself, in the hope that they will leave, or you may feel more confident if you switch on the lights and make a lot of noise by moving about. Even if you are on your own, call out loudly to an imaginary companion; most burglars will flee empty-handed rather than risk a confrontation. Ring the police as soon as it is safe for you to do so. A telephone extension in your bedroom will make you feel more secure as it allows you to call the police immediately, without alerting the intruder.

- Draw your curtains after dark, and if you think there is a prowler outside dial 999.
- Use only your surname and initials in the telephone directory and on the doorplate. That way a stranger won't know if a male or female lives there.
- If you see signs of a break-in at your home, like a smashed window or open door, do not go in. Go to a neighbour and call the police.
- When you answer the phone, simply say 'hello'; do not give your number. If the caller claims to have a wrong number, ask him or her to repeat the number required. Never reveal information about yourself to a stranger or say that you are alone in the house.
- If you receive an abusive or threatening phone call, put the receiver down beside the phone, and walk away. Come back a few minutes later and replace the receiver; do not listen to see if the caller is still there. Do not say anything: an emotional reaction is just what the caller wants. This allows the caller to say what he or she wants to say, without causing distress to you. If the calls continue, tell the police and the operator and keep a record of the date, time and content of each phone call. This may help the authorities trace the caller.

11 Ways in which men can help

- Men can help by taking the issue of women's safety seriously and bearing the following points in mind:
- If you are walking in the same direction as a woman who is on her own, do not walk behind her as this may worry her. Cross the road and walk on the other side. This may reassure her that you are not following her.
- Do not sit too close to a woman on her own in a railway carriage or bus. If you are thinking of chatting to a woman waiting, for example, at a lonely bus stop, remember that she won't know you mean no harm.
- Realize how threatening actions such as staring, whistling, passing comments and jostling can be, particularly if you are one of a group of men.
- Help female friends or family members by giving them a lift or walking them home when you can. If you do, make sure they are safely indoors before you leave.

12 Ways in which women can help

- Women can help by taking the issue of personal safety seriously and bearing the following points in mind:

- Always try to plan ahead.
- Always make someone aware of your movements.
- Don't make yourself a target.
- Follow these tips and turn them into habitual behaviour.

Adopting and internalizing these simple precautions can minimize risk and maximize your personal safety.

BE SAFE and STAY SAFE

Principles of health and safety at work

Though we can argue that there was probably a need much earlier, the recognition of a need for explicit guidelines and legislation governing health and safety at work only became readily apparent during the Industrial Revolution, as a consequence of increased industrial activity and production.

Today the principles of health and safety at work are based on the Health and Safety at Work Act (1974), amended in 1986. Regulations made under this Act apply to all work activities in any area of employment, though there are many aspects that relate specifically to health care and the working environment of a busy hospital and other health care settings.

The main objectives of this Act are to:

- ensure the health, safety and well-being of people whilst at work
- protect those not working from the dangers associated with work-related activity
- control and monitor the use of substances hazardous to health
- regulate and monitor the release of toxic substances into the atmosphere.

There are three main organizations responsible for the implementation of this Act. These are:

1 The Health and Safety Commission, who propose new policies, review current policy and promote the objectives of the Act.
2 The Health and Safety Executive, who make arrangements for enforcement of legislation and also provide an Employment Medical Advisory Service. The latter offers advice on health at work and a confidential telephone information service that workers can call for individual guidance or to report a health and safety problem within the workplace.
3 The Health and Safety Inspectorate, who inspect most workplaces, ensuring that health and safety regulations are maintained and implemented.

There are also a number of other organizations related specifically to health care whose aim is to protect and promote public health and safety, the most notable being:

National Client Safety Agency

AIM: to encourage staff to report incidents without fear of personal repri-mand in order that risks are reported. Risks are identified and solutions developed to prevent reoccurrence.

Marble Arch Tower
55 Bryanston Street
London
W1H 7AJ
Tel: 020 7868 2203
www.enquiries@npsa.org.uk

Medical Devices Agency

AIM: to take all reasonable steps to protect the public health and safeguard the interests of clients and users by ensuring that medical devices and equipment meet appropriate standards of safety, quality and performance and that they all comply with relevant European Union Directives.

Hannibal House
Elephant & Castle
London
SE1 6TQ
Tel: 020 7972 8000
www.mail@medical-devices.gov.uk

Medicines Control Agency

AIM: to protect and promote high standards of public health through the regulation of the quality, efficacy and safety of human medicine.

Market Towers
1 Nine Elms Lane
London
SW8 5NQ
Tel: 020 7273 0000
www.info@mca.qsi.gov.uk

But who is responsible for health and safety? The answer is simply all of us.

The Act states that employers must 'safeguard, as far as is reasonably practicable, the health, safety and welfare of their employees', and it is an employer's duty to ensure that employees are aware of any changes at work that may affect health and safety and how to manage risks appro-priately, for example moving/handling or fire.

Employees have a duty to 'take reasonable care' to avoid injury to themselves and others. It is therefore the responsibility of employees to co-operate with the employer, taking care of their own health and safety, that of those around them and those who might be affected by their actions such as clients, relatives, visitors and colleagues. This includes using work items correctly, as instructed; maintaining training and education related to health and safety; and not interfering with, or misusing, anything provided to assist in the implementation of health and safety practices.

It is the responsibility of clients and visitors to adhere to any health and safety instructions in force in the health care setting, for example switching off mobile phones or paying attention to wet-floor cones.

Within most clinical practice areas there are local policies, procedures and guideline documents based on many of the objectives of the Health and Safety at Work Act (1974). Whilst some documents are there to provide guidance for staff members, some form policies that are a condition of employment. Each and every member of staff is personally responsible for ensuring that they regularly read and adhere to the policies within their sphere of practice and attend mandatory updates as required by their employer and regulatory body.

It is essential that all staff working in the health care arena are familiar with the policies and procedures in relation to the following specific areas.

Control of Substances Hazardous to Health (COSHH)

Control of Substances Hazardous to Health are regulations that have been developed by the Health and Safety Executive (1999b) and which require employers to control the exposure of staff, clients and others to hazardous substances. Within the health care setting this includes cleaning agents and disinfectants; heavy metals such as mercury; anaesthetic gases; medicines including cytotoxic drugs; ionizing radiation; the potential risks associated with blood and body fluids; and issues surrounding general bacterial contamination. COSHH regulations are enforceable under the Health and Safety at Work Act and employers can be prosecuted for failure to comply with the regulations.

COSHH requirements include:

- assessing the risk
- deciding what precautions are needed
- preventing or controlling the risk
- ensuring control measures are used and maintained
- monitoring exposure
- informing and instructing employees.

Ionizing radiation protection

Ionizing radiation is frequently used in acute care settings to establish disability or deformity, for example fractures in the form of X-rays. It is also used extensively in investigative procedures, for example CT scanning, and can sometimes form the basis of treatment, such as radiotherapy. Wherever staff, clients and visitors are – or are at risk of being – exposed to radioactive substances the employer is beholden to provide guidelines to staff to ensure safety. Equally staff have an obligation to attend mandatory training and familiarize themselves with all health and safety regulations pertinent to their area of practice. The area of greatest concern to all members of the health care team are the risks associated with blood and body fluids. The following sections outline the universally agreed precautions, though the reader is reminded at this juncture to also consult local policies and procedures.

Universal precautions

Universal precautions are based on the assumption that all blood and body fluids are a possible source of infection, and as such describe systems of safe practice aimed at:

- reducing the risk of cross-infection to and from clients and staff members
- maintaining the confidentiality of known carriers of infections
- reducing the level of contact that staff have with blood and body fluids.

Responsibilities

As stated above, employers are responsible for ensuring that the working environment is maintained in such a way as to minimize risk, and that regulations are adhered to. In relation to universal precautions, this includes the immunization and education of staff, the provision of adequate staffing levels, making contemporary, evidence-based guidelines readily available, and providing:

- handwashing facilities
- sharps containers
- protective clothing, for example masks and gloves
- disposal bags for infected waste
- adequate cleaning materials and equipment.

Health care workers have a legal and professional responsibility to effectively utilize these provisions.

Whilst copies of hospital guidelines are usually found within each individual unit or clinical area it remains the responsibility of the employee to read these, apply them to practice and assess the potential risks involved with all activities. Support is available within most clinical areas from specialist infection control teams, who provide advice and support for clients, staff and relatives in relation to infection management.

Let us now look at each provision in turn, noting its importance and utilization.

Handwashing

Cross-infection, that is, the spread of infection from one person or area to another, is often caused through direct hand contact. Resident bacteria are present in the deep layers of the skin on the hands and, whilst difficult to remove by handwashing, have a low potential to cause infection.

Transient bacteria, on the other hand, have a shorter lifespan but can pass easily from one person to another and have been found to be responsible for the majority of hospital-acquired infections. Effective techniques for washing hands are sufficient to remove most of these bacteria and thus radically reduce the potential for and incidence of cross-infection, yet numerous studies inform us that hospital staff do not undertake the activity either regularly or effectively (EPIC 2001).

Hospital-acquired infections – infections passed from one person to another whilst in hospital – also known as nosocomial infections, can cause deterioration in health, prolong hospital admissions and even lead to death, as well as affecting clients' overall well-being. They therefore impact not only on clients and their families but also on the health service and staff through increases in spending, longer waiting lists and the potential for future litigation. Indeed some infections have now become resistant to all available treatments; it is therefore crucial that their spread be prevented.

In acknowledging this problem, which currently costs the Health Service in excess of £21 million per year, the Department of Health (2001) has published benchmark standards for reducing the number of hospital-acquired infections. This document states that hands should be washed before and after every client contact or activity that may contaminate the hands.

Prior to washing the hands some general points to consider include:

- The removal of all jewellery. Most hospital policies allow staff to wear a plain band wedding ring whilst working in the health care setting but no other jewellery, including wristwatches. This reduces the risk of bacteria being harboured beneath such items, reduces the risk of accident or injury in the workplace and facilitates good handwashing technique.

- Any abrasions or cuts should be covered with an occlusive, waterproof dressing. This reduces the risk of cross-infection thus protecting staff and clients.
- Fingernails should be short and filed smooth, to reduce the risk of accident or injury to client or staff and to reduce the risk of harbouring infection.
- Skin should be well moisturized, reducing the risk of skin dryness and damage and thus reducing the potential for harbouring bacteria.

Handwashing procedure

The purpose of handwashing is to remove resident bacteria and thus reduce the risk of cross-infection.

Equipment

The equipment needed comprises hot and cold running water, appropriate cleansing agent, paper towels and a waste bin (preferably foot operated). The procedures and rationales are given below.

Procedure	Rationale
Roll up sleeves (if applicable) and remove jewellery/wristwatch (if worn)	To promote thorough washing of areas where bacteria can accumulate
Turn on taps and regulate temperature. The water should be hot but comfortable	Hot water improves the efficacy of the cleansing agent, but ensure safety – do not scald
Wet hands and wrists thoroughly	Aids dispersion of cleaning agent
Dispense cleaning agent from dispenser, apply enough agent to produce lather	For effective cleaning, covering all surfaces
Do not use bars of soap	Soap bars can harbour bacteria
Wash hands • using friction on all surfaces • rub palms together • hand-over-hand washing between the fingers • wash fingertips in the palm of each hand, rubbing the palms also • wash fingertips and nails individually • wash thumbs and wrists • wash beneath wedding ring if worn • pay attention to non-dominant hand	To clean effectively all areas paying attention to those frequently missed, e.g. thumbs, between fingers, fingertips and wrists Non-dominant hand is often not washed as well as the dominant hand, therefore pay greater attention to this hand

Procedure	Rationale
The use of nail brushes is not generally recommended	Nail brushes can damage the skin and therefore increase the infection risk
Rinse hands under tolerably hot running water, with hands held downwards, until all cleaning agent removed	Promotes the removal of residual cleaning agent and bacteria. Any residual cleaning agent may cause irritation to the skin
Turn off taps using elbow tap, or use a paper towel if standard tap	Ideally 'elbow' taps should be used to prevent recontamination from touching the tap. If standard tap in use, a clean paper towel should be used to turn off the tap to prevent recontamination
Dry hands thoroughly with clean disposable paper towels	Bacteria flourish in moist areas. Hot air dryers do not dry effectively and communal towels are generally contaminated from previous use
Dry from fingertip upwards	Reduces the risk of recontamination from the forearms
Dispose of paper towel in foot-operated bin	Prevents recontamination from touching bin. If hand-operated, use a clean paper towel to protect hand whilst opening, as with taps
Apply hand cream but avoid using communal tubes or bottles as these have been found to promote cross-infection	Reduces the potential for cracking and splitting

Sharps

What are sharps? Sharps are any item that may cut or penetrate the skin. Within the clinical setting these include:

- surgical instruments
- puncture points on intravenous fluid administration sets
- glass medication ampoules
- needles
- lancets.

One can clearly identify the potential risk for injury and cross-infection where sharp items are concerned and this relates not only to the person using the equipment but also to other team members who are involved in the disposal of used equipment such as porters.

Most injuries involving sharps could be avoided. It is the responsibility of each individual to help reduce this risk by adhering to the following points for the safe use and disposal of sharps.

The points of practice for the safe use and disposal of sharps are given below.

Procedure	Rationale
The individual using the sharp(s) is accountable for safe disposal, and should therefore be aware of the exact type and number of sharps being used and account for the disposal of each item following completion of the procedure	To ensure safety of self and others. Take the sharps bin with you and dispose of the sharp(s) at the point of use/site of task. To reduce the risk of injury to user or others whilst transporting the used equipment and to ensure that staff dispose of equipment immediately and do not leave used sharps around the clinical area
Never re-sheath a needle	Resheathing needles increases the risk of needlestick injury
Dispose of needles and syringes as a complete unit	This reduces the risk of needlestick injury and minimizes the risk of coming into contact with any remaining contaminated fluids within the syringe or sharps container
Always dispose of sharps into an approved container	To reduce the risk of injury and to ensure the safe transportation, disposal and incineration of used equipment
Never fill sharps containers more than two-thirds full, and then lock the seal	Overfilling prevents adequate closure and increases the risk of spillage and injury
Keep sharps boxes out of reach of children, confused clients or those likely to abuse the contents	To reduce the risk of injury and cross-infection. Most sharps boxes are brightly coloured and tempting to the young or confused client or visitor. Some clients/visitors may be tempted to reuse contents, e.g. needles
Do not use sharps containers to dispose of any other materials, e.g. packaging, swabs	Disposal of sharps containers is very expensive compared to the cost entailed in disposing of ordinary or other clinical waste

Remember: gloves do not protect against a sharps injury. Be vigilant at all times

Sharps injury

In the event of a sharps injury it is essential that you adhere to the procedures given below.

Procedure	Rationale
Encourage bleeding from the wound	To help expel any foreign micro-organisms
Do not suck or rub the injury	Sucking will simply transfer the organism into your mouth and rubbing will assist in dispersion of the organism into the bloodstream and surrounding tissue
Wash the area thoroughly with soap and water	To help remove micro-organisms and clean the surrounding tissue to reduce the risk of infection
Cover the injury with an occlusive waterproof dressing	To reduce the risk of further infection and to protect others from cross-infection
Inform Occupational Health	They will document the incident in your personal records and arrange a blood sample for baseline tests should you develop any illness in future. If the client is known or thought to be HIV positive, post-exposure prophylaxis (PEP) may be required. This is a combination of anti-viral drugs needs to be given within one hour of the incident. It is therefore essential that you are aware of and follow this procedure immediately following injury
Inform your line manager and complete the appropriate documentation	To ensure that the injury is reported and facilitates further risk assessment by your ward manager and those charged with the responsibility for risk assessment and management. Fully documenting the incident also provides evidence should there be any future investigation into the incident. Further information can be obtained from your local occupational health service

Protective clothing

It is the responsibility of the employer to provide staff with protective clothing and it is the responsibility of employees to use this equipment correctly.

One aim of the universal precautions is to reduce the level of contact staff have with blood and body fluids. Body fluids refer to urine, faeces, vomit, saliva, vaginal secretions, amniotic fluid, breast milk, semen, and peritoneal, cerebrospinal and synovial fluid.

We can reduce the level of contact with these fluids by the use of:

- **Gloves** - staff should always wear gloves when the risk of coming into contact with a client's blood or body fluids is high. The make of gloves available in the clinical setting tends to vary as suppliers compete for business. The range, however, usually includes plastic/latex gloves that have been powdered, and powder-free gloves. Some may be sterile whilst others are considered socially clean. The activity to be undertaken should dictate whether or not gloves are necessary; in other words, what is the risk of coming into contact with blood and/or body fluid? It is the responsibility of the individual to assess the risks involved and, if deemed necessary, to select the most appropriate gloves. However, sterile gloves should always be worn for any invasive procedures, to reduce the risk of cross-infection. **Remember:** hands are not clean merely because gloves are worn. Regular effective handwashing is still essential before and after using gloves.

- **Aprons** - disposable plastic or water-repellent aprons must be worn when at risk of contamination by blood or body fluids. It is also recommended that staff use aprons to minimize cross-infection when performing routine tasks such as bed making. Aprons are usually colour coded within hospital settings, white aprons being used for most day-to-day clinical activities and yellow or green aprons used when handling food. It is important that you familiarize yourself with local policy.

- **Masks** - facemasks should be worn if there is a risk of splashes of blood or body fluids to the face. Special respiratory masks are sometimes used when caring for specific client groups, for example clients with TB or where clients are immunosuppressed.

- **Eye protection** - should be used when there is a risk of body fluids or blood splashing into the eyes as might occur during childbirth, paracentesis or obtaining cerebrospinal fluid for example.

Should an accident occur involving the eyes or mouth the procedure outlined below should be adhered to strictly.

Procedure	Rationale
Eyes Irrigate with copious amounts of water or 0.9 per cent sodium chloride for at least five minutes	To clean the eye and remove remaining contaminated fluid
Inform Occupational Health immediately	To report incident, for health check and further advice. Post-exposure prophylaxis may be required

Procedure	Rationale
Eyes (continued) Inform your line manager and complete appropriate documentation	To ensure that the injury is reported and facilitate further risk assessment by your ward manager and those charged with the responsibility for risk assessment and management. Fully documenting the incident also provides evidence should there be any future investigation into the incident
Mouth Rinse the mouth thoroughly with water or 0.9 per cent normal saline for at least five minutes but **do not swallow**	To remove remaining contaminated fluid and prevent ingestion of contaminated fluid
Inform Occupational Health immediately	To report incident, undergo health check and obtain further advice
Inform line manager and complete appropriate documentation	To ensure that the injury is reported and facilitate further risk assessment by your ward manager and those charged with the responsibility for risk assessment and management. Fully documenting the incident also provides evidence should there be any future investigation into the incident

Further information can be obtained from the local occupational health service.

Spillages of blood or body fluids *must* be cleaned up promptly. The procedure outlined below should be adhered to strictly.

Procedure	Rationale
Place wet-floor warning sign over area	To reduce risk of accidental slippage on wet floor
Wear disposable gloves and apron	To protect against contamination and reduce the risk of cross-infection
Absorb liquid using paper towels, and dispose into yellow clinical waste bag at site	To remove excess and limit spread of contaminated fluid to one area

Procedure	Rationale
Mop floor using hot soapy water and designated mop	To remove all contaminated liquid and prevent cross-infection
Rinse out the mop and send mop head to laundry for cleaning as per local policy	To decontaminate
In the case of blood spillages only Apply 1% sodium hypochlorite solution or sprinkle with disinfectant granules and leave for several minutes before following the above procedure	Recommended cleaning agent for blood spillages; needs to be left to absorb fluid

Disposal of clinical waste

Linen

Any linen that is soiled with blood or body fluid or deemed infected should be placed in a water-soluble bag and then placed inside the appropriate laundry bag depending on local policy. Some hospitals use yellow laundry bags for infected linen and red for linen contaminated with blood or body fluids. Be sure to familiarize yourself with your local policy and procedure.

The notion of 'double bagging' laundry is to protect laundry staff who can then transfer soiled linen into the washing machines without having to handle the contaminated contents.

Waste bags

- Yellow bags – used for the disposal of any waste arising from direct client care, for example soiled clinical dressings, swabs or containers.
- Black bags – used for the disposal of normal household waste such as paper towels.
- Brown paper bags or boxes – used for the disposal of glass and aerosols.
- White plastic or clear bags – used to return used reusable items to the sterile supplies department for re-sterilization.

Note: it is far more expensive to incinerate clinical waste than to dispose of household waste in a landfill site. It is the responsibility of all staff to dispose of waste appropriately, to maintain the health and safety of other workers and to consider the environmental and financial costs involved.

Principles of asepsis

Asepsis means freedom from pathogenic (that is, disease-causing) micro-organisms, whilst sepsis indicates the presence of micro-organisms causing toxicity in the body. Infection can occur endogenously or exogenously.

- **Endogenous** – from sites on or in the host, for example from the client's skin, nose, or intestines
- **Exogenous** – from routes outside the host or environmental, such as:
  - airborne, for example droplets, dust, dressings, bedding
  - direct or indirect contact, for example hands, clothing, equipment, and food
  - percutaneously, for example intravenous infusions, needles.

In order to reduce the potential for exogenous infection, nurses and other health care professionals employ what is termed a sterile (or aseptic), non-touch technique when undertaking invasive procedures such as urethral catheterization and injections, or procedures where the risk of cross-infection is high, for example when dressing wounds or removing sutures and drains. The basic principles of this technique are outlined below.

Aseptic or non-touch technique

The main aim of this technique is to reduce the risk of cross-infection or contamination during clinical procedures. The equipment required will be dependent upon the task but generally includes a dressing trolley or other clean working surface, sterile gloves, disposable apron, sterile dressing pack, sterile forceps (if required), sterile fluids, syringe and receptacle (if necessary), appropriate dressing(s) and hypo-allergenic tape. The procedure is outlined below.

Procedure	Rationale
Explain procedure to the client, ensure adequate understanding and obtain consent	To gain informed consent and ensure co-operation
Encourage the client to adopt an appropriate and comfortable position and loosen dressing(s) without exposing the patient unduly	To reduce anxiety, promote comfort and facilitate ease of procedure whilst maintaining dignity

Procedure	Rationale
Prepare the environment and allow airborne dust and micro-organisms to settle before proceeding	To reduce the potential for cross-infection
Put on appropriate plastic apron and wash hands thoroughly (see above)	To reduce the risk of cross-infection and to remove transient organisms
Clean dressing trolley with alcoholic surface wipe or soap and water if debris evident, cleaning from top to bottom and drying thoroughly (refer to local policy)	To provide a clean working surface. Washing from top to bottom moves any micro-organisms down from the work surface and reduces the likelihood of recontamination
Collect all equipment and place on bottom shelf of trolley	Maintains a clean empty work surface
Take trolley/equipment to the client, disturbing the area as little as possible	To minimize airborne contamination
Check the expiry date on sterile dressing pack; make sure it is intact and dry. Open the outer cover of the pack and slide the contents onto the trolley top	To ensure that only sterile products are used
Open sterile field/paper using corners only and position over work surface	To reduce the risk of contamination and to provide a sterile working area
Position contents of pack then check and open any other packages, maintaining sterility of field	To ensure all equipment is sterile and readily accessible
Remove soiled dressing(s) using forceps	To reduce risk of contamination
Wash hands thoroughly using appropriate cleaning agent	To reduce risk of cross-contamination
If using sterile gloves apply now, touching only the inside of the cuff	To maintain sterility of glove. Gloves allow greater dexterity for user and reduce risk of further trauma for client
Place sterile field around area, e.g. wound, perineum	To provide a sterile working area in close proximity to area requiring cleaning or dressing and to reduce the risk of contamination
Cleanse the wound if necessary	Wounds only require cleaning if infected, and should be irrigated rather than swabbed, to reduce the likelihood of tissue damage. Clean wounds should always be dressed first to reduce the potential for cross-infection

Procedure	Rationale
Apply and secure dressing as appropriate, ensuring client comfort	To protect the wound, promote healing and ensure client compliance
Dispose of clinical waste and instruments as per universal precautions and hospital policy	To reduce risk of contamination to others or environment
Dispose of apron and gloves, if worn, in appropriate receptacle	To reduce the risk of cross-infection
Wash and dry dressing trolley	To reduce the risk of cross-infection
Wash hands thoroughly	To reduce the risk of cross-infection
Document care given and report any changes or abnormalities in evaluation	Legal requirement to maintain documentation and safeguard client through effective communication

Monitoring a client's pulse

The pulse is a wave of pressure produced by the expansion of an artery due to contraction of the left ventricle of the heart.

The pulse can be felt with the fingertips at the following points:

- temporal – the temple
- carotid – the side of the neck
- brachial – the antecubital fossa (crook) of the arm
- radial – in the wrist below the thumb
- femoral – in the groin
- popliteal – behind the knee
- posterior tibial – to the side of the ankle
- dorsalis pedis – on the front of the foot.

Other terminology used when monitoring the pulse include:

- tachycardia – a pulse above the normal range
- bradycardia – a pulse below the normal range.

Many factors influence the pulse and these include:

- age
- gender
- physique
- body temperature

- haemorrhage
- exercise
- stress
- some prescribed medications, for example digoxin, tricyclic antidepressants, caffeine, nicotine, alcohol
- some illegal substances, for example ecstasy.

Assessing the pulse

Monitoring a client's pulse forms part of the assessment of vital signs and assists nursing and medical staff in determining the client's general health and well-being. The equipment needed comprises a watch with a second hand and an appropriate chart for recording. The procedures are outlined below.

Procedure	Rationale
Explain procedure and obtain consent	To gain informed consent and reduce anxiety
Wash hands thoroughly	To minimize the risk of cross-infection
Place fingertips over selected artery, apply gentle pressure and feel for pulse	To confirm position and identify pulse. If you apply too much pressure you may occlude the blood supply and therefore you will not be able to feel the pulse
Begin to count pulse and, using a watch, follow the sweeping second hand for 60 seconds	To elicit the rate

Normal ranges (beats per minute):
    Newborn: 70-190
    2-5 years: 80-160
    6-14 years: 70-120
    Adult: 55-90
Note the rhythm (pattern) of the beats
	To determine intervals between each beat and check the regularity. Any abnormal rhythm (arrhythmia) should be reported immediately

Record on appropriate chart (see Figure 4.1) and/or care plan and report any deviation in rate, rhythm or strength	Legal requirement to maintain documentation and safeguard client through good communications
Wash hands thoroughly	To reduce risk of cross-infection

Figure 4.1 Example of a care plan

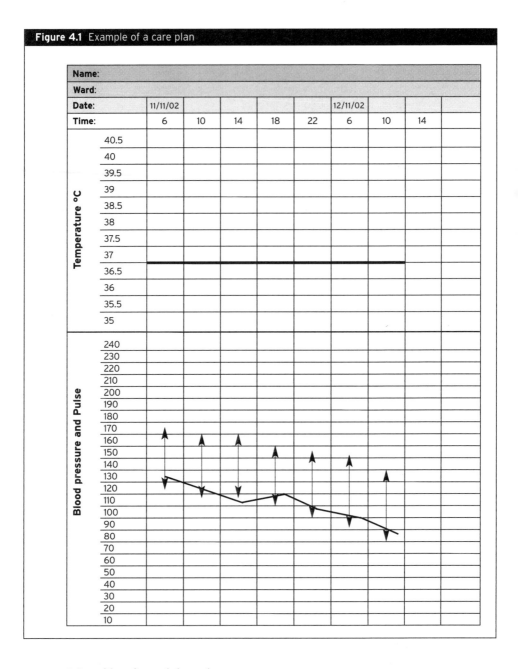

Name:									
Ward:									
Date:	11/11/02					12/11/02			
Time:	6	10	14	18	22	6	10	14	

Monitoring blood pressure

Blood pressure is the pressure exerted on resisting artery walls as blood is forced through from the heart.

Monitoring a client's blood pressure measurements helps nursing and medical staff to establish the ability of the client's arteries to fill with blood, the efficiency of the heart as a pump, and the volume of circulating blood. It is normally taken using the arm but the thigh can also be used if required.

There are two types of blood pressure:

- systolic - the highest pressure reached during contraction of the heart
- diastolic - the pressure remaining in the ventricles when the heart is resting between contractions

Factors that may influence blood pressure include:

- high body temperature
- exposure to heat/cold
- stress
- obesity
- smoking
- alcohol
- heart disease
- haemorrhage.

Blood pressure measurement

Monitoring a client's blood pressure forms part of the assessment of vital signs and assists nursing and medical staff in determining the client's cardiovascular status, general health and well-being. The only pieces of equipment needed are an appropriate device and a stethoscope (if required).

It is recommended that you use an electronic device for infants and children as the pulse is generally difficult to hear. The most commonly used devices are:

- manual mercury sphygmomanometer, which measures blood pressure using mercury
- manual aneroid sphygmomanometer, which measures blood pressure using air
- electronic automated devices, which measure the sound of the blood as it passes through the artery, and then display the pressure on a monitor.

All the devices measure in millimetres of mercury, usually expressed as mmHg.

Remember, machines can and do malfunction; if the reading seems too high or low given the client's overall condition and demeanour recheck the measurement either by using another machine or by checking it manually. All devices should be inspected and calibrated annually.

The procedures are outlined below.

Procedure	Rationale
Explain procedure and ensure adequate understanding	To ensure informed consent and obtain client's co-operation
Before proceeding check that the client is rested, and has not been consuming alcohol or nicotine, and advise them not to talk during the procedure	To ensure an accurate reading
Ensure client is positioned correctly	To ensure accuracy of reading. Blood pressure readings should be taken in the same position and on the same limb each time if possible. The dominant side is recommended if at all possible. It is therefore good practice to document position to ensure continuity of care, e.g. lying, standing, sitting, and whether you have used the left or right limb. In some instances it may be necessary to record both lying and standing blood pressure, in which case it is important to distinguish between the two as per local preferences
Ensure correct-size cuff	Correct cuff size must be used for accurate reading. Size and instructions are usually printed on the inside of cuff
Apply the cuff 2.5 cm above the ante-cubital fossa with the client's palm upwards, ensuring that the cuff is level with the sphygmomanometer and the client's heart	To ensure accuracy of reading. Inaccurate readings occur if equipment is not in correct alignment. **NB** Do not use a limb receiving intravenous therapy and make sure that clothing above the cuff is not restrictive otherwise the accuracy of the reading will be questionable
If using an automated device commence the reading	This reading provides a rough estimate of the systolic blood pressure and reduces the possible discomfort arising from hyper inflation of the cuff
If undertaking the measurement manually, locate the radial pulse on the cuffed arm then inflate the cuff until the pulse is no longer felt - note the point at which this happens on the sphygmomanometer scale	
Deflate the cuff for 30 seconds ensuring that all air has been released	To allow circulation to return to the limb

Procedure	Rationale
Locate the brachial artery and place the stethoscope over the pulse	Locating the artery prior to inflating the cuff ensures that the strongest point of the pulse can be identified and heard during the reading
Inflate the cuff again to approximately 20–30mmHg above the estimated systolic reading	To apply pressure to the artery in order to then hear and record the blood pressure
Deflate the cuff, slowly, at approximately 2–3mmHg per second and **listen**	Whilst slow deflation may be uncomfortable for the client, deflating too quickly will not allow time to hear the blood pressure sounds and mean that the procedure has to be repeated
Listen for and note the first sound that you hear (systolic); this will be followed by the other sounds listed. Note the point at which the sound disappears (diastolic)	To the attuned, five different sounds can be heard, known as Korotkoff sounds: 1 The first clear tapping sound = systolic 2 A swishing sound 3 An intense clear tap 4 A muffled sound 5 Sounds disappear altogether = diastolic
Compare reading with client's previous reading and normal range and note any abnormality or improvement. If necessary repeat the reading but allow the client to rest the limb between attempts	Normal range: Newborn 80/40 mmHg 1–7 years 100/65 mmHg 8–12 years 100/70 mmHg Adult 120/80 mmHg Elderly systolic 100 + age In the elderly the diastolic may rise also
Record blood pressure measurement on appropriate documentation (see Figure 4.1) and report any abnormalities	Legal requirement to maintain documentation and safeguard client through effective communications
Remove and clean equipment	To reduce the risk of cross-infection. **NB** Automated machines should not be used on clients being nursed in isolation
Wash hands thoroughly	

Responding in the event of a cardiopulmonary arrest

A cardiopulmonary arrest, that is, a situation where the client is pulseless and not breathing, requires an urgent and well-trained response. It is therefore essential that all health care personnel receive initial training in basic life support (BLS) and attend regular updates, at least annually, to maintain their skills.

Basic life support involves an initial assessment followed by airway maintenance, rescue breathing and chest compressions, the word 'basic' suggesting that no equipment is used. Where a simple airway or facemask for mouth-to-mouth ventilation is used, this is termed 'basic life support with airway adjunct'. The purpose of BLS is to maintain adequate ventilation and circulation until such time as the primary cause of the cardiac arrest can be addressed and, where possible, corrected. It is important to remember that failure of circulation to the brain for 3–4 minutes (less if the client is already hypoxaemic) will lead to irreversible brain damage. Immediate recognition and commencement of BLS is therefore crucial, as any delay will lessen the client's chance of recovery.

The three elements of basic life support after initial assessment are commonly remembered as 'ABC': *Airway, Breathing and Circulation*.

The following procedures have been developed from the Resuscitation Council UK (2000) Basic Life Support Resuscitation Guidelines with the kind permission of the Vice-Chairman of the Council.

Sequence of actions for adult BLS

For the purposes of these guidelines an adult is considered to be any individual 8 years of age or older. The male pronoun has been used for ease of reading.

If you are alone:	
Check that it is safe to approach, ensuring safety of rescuer and client	To prevent injury to self
Check the client and see if he responds. Gently shake his shoulders and ask loudly: 'Are you all right?'	To ensure that the client has not merely fainted
If he responds by answering or moving leave him in the position in which you find him (provided he is not in further danger), check his condition, get assistance if needed and reassess him regularly	
If he does not respond shout for help	To alert others and to increase the client's chances of recovery

If you are alone:

Unless you can assess the client fully in the position you find him, turn him onto his back and open his airway by placing your hand on his forehead and gently tilting his head back, keeping your thumb and index finger free to close his nose if rescue breathing is required

Remove any visible obstruction from the client's mouth, including any dislodged dentures. Leave well-fitting dentures in place, and, with your fingertips under the tip of the client's chin, lift the chin to open the airway. Avoid tilting the head if injury to the neck is suspected

To open the airway
Well-fitting dentures can assist in obtaining a seal

To avoid further injury (see 'Cervical spine injury')

Keeping the airway open, look, listen and feel for breathing (as described in Chapter 1)

To ensure absence of breathing

If he **is** breathing normally turn him into the recovery position (see Chapter 2) and send or go for help. Check for continued breathing

To maintain airway

If the client is **not** breathing or is only making occasional gasps or weak attempts at breathing send someone for help or, if you are on your own, leave the client and go for help. On return start rescue breathing as described in Chapter 1. Do not make more than five attempts in all to achieve two effective breaths. Even if unsuccessful, move on to assessment of the circulation

To ensure that others are alerted

Failure to restore circulation if absent will increase the potential for cerebral damage

Assess the client for signs of a circulation. Only if you have been trained to do so, check the carotid pulse, taking no more than 10 seconds to do this

To ascertain whether cardiac massage is required

If you are confident that you have detected signs of circulation continue rescue breathing until the client starts breathing on his own. About every 10 breaths (or about every minute) recheck for signs of a circulation; take no more than 10 seconds each time. If the client starts to breathe normally on his own but remains unconscious, turn him into the recovery position. Be ready to turn him on to his back and restart rescue breathing if he stops breathing

To maintain oxygenation

To maintain airway

If there are no signs of a circulation, or you are at all unsure, start chest compressions. With your hand that is nearest the client's feet, locate the lower half of the sternum (breastbone)

To restore circulation

If you are alone:

Using your index and middle fingers, identify the lower rib edge nearest to you. Keeping your fingers together, slide them upwards to the point where the ribs join the sternum. With your middle finger on this point, place your index finger on the sternum itself.

Slide the heel of your other hand down the sternum until it reaches your index finger; this should be the middle of the lower half of the sternum.

Place the heel of the other hand on top of the first.

Extend or interlock the fingers of both hands and lift them to ensure that pressure is not applied over the client's ribs.

Do not apply any pressure over the upper abdomen or bottom tip of the sternum.

Position yourself vertically above the client's chest and, with your arms straight, press down on the sternum to depress it 4-5 cm.

Release all the pressure without losing contact between the hand and sternum, then repeat at a rate of about 100 times a minute (a little less than two compressions a second); it may be helpful to count aloud. Compression and release should take an equal amount of time

| | To prevent further injury and ensure that pressure is applied in the most effective place |

Combine rescue breathing and chest compression. After 15 compressions tilt the head, lift the chin, and give two effective breaths

| | To oxygenate the blood |

Return your hands without delay to the correct position on the sternum and give 15 further compressions, continuing compressions and breaths in a ratio of 15:2

| | Only stop to recheck for signs of circulation if the client makes a movement or takes a spontaneous breath; otherwise resuscitation should not be interrupted |

Continue resuscitation until: qualified help arrives and takes over; **or** the client shows signs of life; **or** you become exhausted

Resuscitation with two persons: Two-person cardiopulmonary resuscitation (CPR) is less tiring than single-person CPR. However, it is important that both rescuers are proficient and practised in the technique. It is therefore recommended that this technique is only used by trained healthcare providers and those lay persons who are members of trained teams, such as first aid and rescue organizations.

- Summon help: this may mean that one rescuer has to start CPR alone whilst the other leaves to find a telephone.
- A ratio of 15 compressions to 2 inflations should be used. By the end of each series of 15 compressions, the rescuer responsible for ventilation should be positioned ready to give 2 inflations with the least possible delay. It is helpful if the rescuer giving compressions counts out aloud. It is preferable that the rescuers work from opposite sides of the client.
- Chin lift and head tilt should be maintained at all times as in Chapter 1, 'Maintenance of an airway'. Ventilations should take 2 seconds each during which chest compressions should cease. Compressions should be resumed immediately after the second inflation of the chest, waiting only for the rescuer to remove his or her lips from the client's face to maintain patency of airway.
- If the rescuers wish to change places, usually because the one giving compressions becomes tired, this should be undertaken as quickly and smoothly as possible. Resuscitation SHOULD NOT BE INTERRUPTED.

Recovery position for adults

Once circulation and breathing have been restored, it is important to maintain a good airway and ensure that the tongue does not cause obstruction. It is also important to minimize the risk of inhalation of gastric contents.

For this reason the client should be placed in the recovery position (see Chapter 2). This will allow the tongue to fall forward, keeping the airway clear.

- If in situ remove the client's spectacles, to avoid injury and damage.
- Kneel beside the client and make sure that both his legs are straight, to facilitate movement.
- Place the arm nearest to you out at right angles to his body, elbow bent with the hand palm uppermost, to protect the head when the client is turned.
- Bring his far arm across the chest, and hold the back of the hand against the client's cheek nearest to you, to prevent injury.
- With your other hand, grasp the far leg just above the knee and pull it up, keeping the foot on the ground, to facilitate movement.
- Keeping his hand pressed against his cheek, pull on the leg to roll the client towards you onto his side.
- Adjust the upper leg so that both the hip and knee are bent at right angles, to help maintain the position.
- Tilt the head back, to make sure the airway remains open.
- Adjust the hand under the cheek, if necessary, to keep the head tilted.

- Check breathing regularly, to monitor condition.
- Care should be taken to monitor the peripheral circulation of the lower arm, and to ensure that the duration for which there is pressure on this arm is kept to a minimum. If the client has to be kept in the recovery position for more than 30 minutes he should be turned to the opposite side, to reduce the likelihood of pressure sores.

Finally, it must be emphasized that in spite of possible problems during training and in use, it remains beyond doubt that placing the unconscious, breathing client into the recovery position can be life saving.

Variations in cardiopulmonary resuscitation techniques

Mouth-to-nose ventilation

There are several situations in which mouth-to-nose ventilation may be preferable to mouth-to-mouth ventilation:

- if mouth-to-mouth ventilation proves technically difficult, for example because of unusual or absent dentition
- if mouth obstruction cannot be relieved
- during rescue of a client from the water, when one hand is required to support the body and cannot be used to close the nose
- when resuscitation is being carried out by a child whose mouth may not be large enough to seal an adult's mouth.

To carry out mouth-to-nose ventilation:

1 Release the client's nose and close his mouth.
2 Seal your mouth around his nose and blow in steadily as for the mouth-to-mouth technique.
3 Allow his mouth to open to let the breath out.

Cervical spine injury

If spinal cord injury is suspected (for example if the client has sustained a fall, been struck on the head or neck, or has been rescued after diving into shallow water) particular care must be taken during handling and resuscitation to maintain alignment of the head, neck, and chest in the neutral position. A spinal board and/or cervical collar should be used if available.

As hypotension often accompanies spinal cord injury, care should be taken to maintain the client in a horizontal position during rescue.

When opening an airway, head tilt may be employed, but the tilt should be kept to a minimum, that is, just enough to allow unobstructed ventilation or intubation. Jaw thrust (see Figure 1.2) rather than chin lift is preferable. During resuscitation, assistance from others may be required to maintain head, back, and chest alignment if adequate splinting is not available. Remember that successful resuscitation that results in paralysis is tragic, but failure to carry out adequate ventilation in cases of respiratory arrest will result in death (Resuscitation Council UK Guidelines 2000).

Sequence of actions for paediatric BLS

An *infant* is considered to be a child under the age of 1 year whilst a *child* is aged between 1 and 8 years of age. Small children over the age of 8 years may still be treated as for a younger child but may require different techniques to attain adequate chest compression.

In the following sequence a 'child' includes an 'infant' unless otherwise specified

Check that it is safe to approach, ensuring safety of rescuer and client	To ensure safety of rescuer and child
Check the child's responsiveness. Gently stimulate the child and ask loudly: 'Are you all right?'	To make sure that the child has not just fainted
Infants, and children with suspected cervical spinal injuries, should not be shaken	Shaking can cause paralysis and head trauma
If the child responds by answering or moving, leave the child in the position in which you find him (provided he is not in further danger). Check his condition and get help if needed. Reassess him regularly	To monitor condition
If the child does not respond, shout for help. Open the child's airway by tilting his head and lifting his chin	To alert others and to increase the child's chances of recovery

If possible with the child in the position in which you find him, place your hand on the child's forehead and gently tilt his head back.
  At the same time, with your fingertip(s) under the point of the child's chin, lift the chin to open the airway.
  Do not push on the soft tissues under the chin.
  If you have any difficulty in opening the airway, carefully turn the child on to his back and then open the airway as described above
	To maintain airway
	
	This may block the airway

Avoid head tilt if trauma or injury to the neck is suspected	If neck injury is suspected use the jaw thrust method of opening the airway (see Figure 1.2)

Keeping the airway open, look, listen and feel for breathing as described in Chapter 1	To ensure absence of breathing
If the child is breathing normally, turn the child on his side and send or go for help. Check for continued breathing	
If the child is not breathing or is making occasional gasps, carefully remove any obvious airway obstruction as described in Chapter 1. Send for or summon help, then commence rescue breathing (see Chapter 1), remembering to take breaths yourself between rescue breaths	To maximize the oxygen you deliver
While performing the rescue breaths, note any gag or cough response to your action	You may stimulate the child to breathe spontaneously

For an infant
Take a breath and cover the mouth and nasal apertures of the infant with your mouth, making sure you have a good seal. In a larger infant, if the mouth-to-mouth-and-nose method is difficult, try the mouth-to-nose technique. In this, the adult's mouth is placed over the infant's nose and rescue breathing attempted. It may be necessary to close the infant's mouth during rescue breathing to prevent air escaping.
    If you have difficulty achieving an effective breath, the airway may be obstructed.
    Recheck the infant's mouth and remove any obstruction.
    Recheck that the head is in the neutral position and that the neck is not over-extended. The jaw thrust method may be attempted if you are unable to establish an open airway (see Figure 1.2).
    Make up to five attempts in all to achieve at least two effective breaths

Assess the child for signs of a circulation. Look for any movement including swallowing, coughing or breathing (more than an occasional breath)	Failure to restore circulation if absent will increase the potential for cerebral damage

For trained health care providers only: check the pulse
Child – feel for the carotid pulse in the neck.
Infant – feel for the brachial pulse on the inner aspect of the upper arm.
Take no more than 10 seconds to do this

If you are confident that you can detect signs of a circulation (or a pulse over 60 beats per minute if you have been trained to do so) within 10 seconds, continue rescue breathing, if necessary, until the child starts breathing effectively on his own.	To maintain oxygenation
Recheck regularly for signs of a circulation, taking no more than 10 seconds.	To monitor condition
If the child starts to breathe normally on his own but remains unconscious turn him into the recovery position.	To maintain airway
Be ready to turn him onto his back and restart rescue breathing if he stops breathing	
If there are no signs of a circulation, or you are at all unsure (or the pulse rate is very slow – less than 60 beats per minute), start chest compression.	To restore adequate circulation
Combine rescue breathing and chest compression	

For a child

Locate and place the heel of one hand over the lower half of the sternum (breastbone) ensuring that you do not compress on or below the xiphisternum.	To prevent fracture or dislocation
Lift the fingers to ensure that pressure is not applied over the child's ribs.	
Position yourself vertically above the chest and, with your arm straight, press down on the sternum to depress it approximately one-third to one-half of the depth of the child's chest.	To achieve effective compression
Release the pressure, then repeat at a rate of about 100 times a minute.	
After five compressions tilt the head, lift the chin and give one effective breath.	
Return your hand immediately to the correct position on the sternum and give five further compressions.	
Continue compressions and breaths in a ratio of 5:1.	
In children over the age of approximately 8 years, it may be necessary to use the 'adult' two-handed method of chest compression to achieve an adequate depth of compression at a ratio of 15:2	

For an infant and a single or non-professional rescuer

Locate the sternum and place the tips of two fingers, one finger's breadth below an imaginary line joining the infant's nipples.	
With the tips of two fingers, press down on the sternum to depress it approximately one-third to one-half of the infant's chest.	Rationale as for child

Release the pressure, then repeat at a rate of about 100 times a minute.
After five compressions tilt the head, lift the chin and give one effective breath.
Return your hands immediately to the correct position on the sternum and give five further compressions.
Continue compressions and breaths in a ratio of 5:1

Continue resuscitation until the client shows signs of life (spontaneous respiration, pulse), qualified help arrives or you become exhausted

(Resuscitation Council UK Guidelines 2000)

Recovery position for children

An unconscious child whose airway is clear, and who is breathing spontaneously, should be turned on his side into the same recovery position as outlined for adults (see Chapter 2). This prevents the tongue falling back to obstruct the airway and reduces the risk of inhalation of stomach contents.

There are, however, a number of different recovery positions, each of which has its advocates. The important principles to be followed are:

- The child should be in as near a true lateral position as possible with his mouth positioned to allow free drainage of fluid.
- The position should be stable. In an infant this may require the support of a small pillow or rolled-up blanket placed behind the back to maintain the position.
- Any pressure on the chest that impairs breathing should be avoided.
- It should be possible to turn the child onto his side and to return him back easily and safely, paying particular attention to the possibility of cervical spine injury.
- Good observation and access to the airway should be possible.

(Source: Resuscitation Council UK 2000)

Administration of medicines

In practice the term 'medicine' is generally taken to mean any substance used therapeutically in the treatment of disease. The control of supply, storage, prescribing and administration of medicines is governed by the following legislation.

Policy

Medicines Act 1968

This Act controls the licensing, manufacture and distribution of medicines and the registration of retail pharmacies. It also categorizes drugs into three groups:

- prescription only – drugs supplied following instruction from a doctor, dentist or nurse prescriber, for example antidepressants
- non-prescription but pharmacy only – drugs that can be supplied by registered community pharmacies (chemists) but can only be sold in the presence of a pharmacist, for example antihistamines
- general sales list medicines – drugs freely obtainable from retail outlets with no prescription or pharmacist supervision, for example paracetamol.

Misuse of Drugs Act 1971

This Act controls the sale and use of substances likely to cause addiction, referred to as controlled drugs (previously known as Dangerous Drugs). These include opium (heroin) and its alkaloids, along with others such as LSD, ecstasy and amphetamines. The Act divides these drugs into three classes, A, B and C, according to their potential to cause harm. Penalties are applied related to the misuse, possession or trafficking of a drug based on its classification. Class A drugs are considered the most harmful to individuals and society and therefore carry the highest penalties. If a class B drug is prepared for injection it becomes a class A drug and the penalties mirror this change. Class C carries the lightest penalties.

The position of cannabis and ecstasy within this classification are currently under review by the Home Affairs Committee of Members of Parliament.

The Act impedes the misuse of controlled drugs without prohibiting correct usage by health care professionals.

Drugs are further divided into five groups or schedules, which are:

Schedule 1 those that cannot be prescribed, for example LSD, raw opium; they may be used for research but a licence is required from the Home Office

Schedule 2 morpine, diamorphine, pethidine and amphetamines

Schedule 3 hypnotic drugs, for example barbiturates

Schedule 4 non-barbiturate sedatives, for example benzodiazipines

Schedule 5 non-prescription – cough mixtures and simple analgesia, which contain very small amounts of controlled substances, for example codeine linctus.

Storage of medicines

The procedures for the storage of medicines are given below.

Procedure	Rationale
All medications must be stored in locked cupboards, trolleys or fridges when not in use. Trolleys and fridges **must** be secured to the wall	To ensure safety and reduce risk of theft and unauthorized use and to maintain stability of drug through appropriate storage
Controlled drugs must be stored in an inner locked cupboard within a second outer locked cupboard with a readily identifiable red external light	To ensure safety, reduce risk of unauthorized misuse and to ensure adherence with legislation
Keys to controlled drugs cupboard and medicines trolley/cupboards **should** be in the keeping of a first-level registered nurse at all times	To prevent unauthorized misuse
Ensure regular checks of stock made by either senior nurse or pharmacist	To maintain stock and check expiry dates of drug, reducing risk of error or misuse
Prescription pads must be kept in locked cupboard	To prevent unauthorized misuse
All prescriptions and order forms must be kept by the hospital or pharmacy for a period of two years from the date of issue	To enable random auditing and security checks

Prescriptions

There are key points to be aware of when administering medications against a printed or hand-written prescription or prior to requesting medicines for a client to take home. These are set out below.

Procedure	Rationale
Ensure prescription is written in indelible ink	To prevent unauthorized changes to prescription
Check the signature of doctor. If a GP practice then address should be printed in full	Confirming identity of prescriber
Name and address of client	To reduce risk of unauthorized misuse or dispensing errors
Age must be written if a child under 12 years	Legal requirement
Name of drug, dosage and frequency clearly written	To ensure clear identification of drug name and details thus reducing risk of potential errors
Preferably no abbreviations but some Latin abbreviations are deemed acceptable (see Appendix 1)	To reduce the potential for drug errors
No more than 28 days' supply can be dispensed at any one time	To control stocks and amount supplied thus preventing misuse and reducing risks of error
There are restrictions placed on the number of repeat prescriptions a GP can make without seeing the client	To ensure appropriate prescribing

Prior to 1998 only doctors and dentists were allowed to prescribe medicines. Since this time, however, individuals who are registered nurses with a district nursing or health visiting qualification, and who have also undertaken a validated Nurse Prescribing course can prescribe a limited range of preparations (see British Medical Association 2003).

Procedure for the safe administration of medicines

In April 2002 the Nursing and Midwifery Council (NMC 2000a) revised the guidelines for the administration of medicines, and these should be adhered to at *all* times. The following procedure is based on those guidelines and gives the rationale for each element. If ever in doubt remember 'the six Rs'.

- Right drug
- Right dose
- Right route
- Right form
- Right time
- Right client

Also remember to become familiar with your local policies related to the administration of medicines before participating in this procedure (see below).

Procedure	Rationale
Wash and dry hands thoroughly	To reduce the risk of cross-infection
Collect prescription sheet and ensure that the client is available and willing to take any prescribed medications	To gain consent and avoid wastage
Ensure that the prescription is dated, legible and signed by a doctor	To fulfil legal requirements related to drug administration
Prior to administration ensure you are knowledgeable about the drug(s) to be administered. This should include: therapeutic use, normal dosage, routes/ forms (see Table 4.1), potential side effects, contra-indications	To ensure safety and well-being of client and to enable you to identify any errors in prescribing
Confirm identity of client verbally and with identification band against prescription, checking full name, home address, date of birth, age, identification number, RIGHT CLIENT and ensure that the drug has not already been given	To ensure that the correct drug is being administered to the correct client
Check the prescription carefully, ascertaining RIGHT DRUG, DOSE, ROUTE, FORM and TIME	To ensure client safety. **If any errors of prescribing are noticed then withhold the drug and inform the medical officer**
Check client understands the need for the drug and answer any questions he or she may have prior to administration	To ensure that consent is informed
Be familiar with the client's care plan and past medical history	To ensure that only the medications currently required are administered. Knowledge of past medical history assists in identifying contra-indications specific to client

Procedure	Rationale
Select the appropriate medication and for a second time check the drug, route, dose, time, form and co-existing therapies prior to administration	To ensure safe administration of the medication
Check the expiry date of all medications to be administered	To protect the client from harm. Medicines that have expired can be dangerous, as products deteriorate over time. Expired medications should be returned to pharmacy for appropriate disposal
Check that the client is not allergic to the drug or any of its derivatives prior to administration	To protect the client from harm. If the client is allergic inform medical staff without delay to review prescription
Administer the medication in the appropriate form, by the prescribed route, at the correct dosage to the correct client and make sure that they have taken/received it	To fulfil your responsibilities and prevent any untoward occurrences
Following administration of the medication ensure clear, accurate and immediate documentation. This includes refusal of medicines by client or any intentionally withheld drugs	Legal requirement to document treatment and safeguard client through effective communication. **Student nurses or midwives must not administer any drug unsupervised and all signatures must be countersigned by a registered practitioner**
Controlled drugs **must** be checked by two nurses/midwives, one of whom must be registered, and the appropriate additional documentation completed	Legal requirement relating to Misuse of Drugs Regulations 1985 and the Misuse of Drugs (Safe Custody) Regulations 1973
Clear away all equipment and ensure safe storage of medications as per local policy	To adhere to health and safety regulations

If you are unsure about any aspect of the medicines prescribed it is advisable to contact the pharmacy staff, who will be only too happy to advise and guide you.

Table 4.1 Advantages and disadvantages of different routes

Route	Advantages	Disadvantages	Form(s)
Oral (O)/ **Sublingual** (S/L) (under the tongue) **Buccal** (Buc) (between lip and gum)	• Comfortable • Non-invasive • Easy to use • Inexpensive	Cannot use if client has: • Nausea or vomiting • Reduced gut motility, bowel disease or malabsorption • Difficulty swallowing • Impaired consciousness • OR if the client is to remain nil by mouth (NBM)	Tablet Capsule Elixir Gel
Intramuscular injection (I/M)	• Rapid and assured absorption • Effective if client unable to use oral medication • Can sometimes combine drugs into one injection	• More expensive • Client anxiety and discomfort on administration • Increased risk of side effects with rapid absorption • Risk of introducing infection • Risks involved with sharps usage • Slower absorption if client is cold	Single-use glass or plastic vial Liquid solution or powder requiring reconstitution
Subcutaneous injection (S/C)	• Slow sustained absorption • Virtually pain free • Suitable for repeated injections or infusion	• Risk of ulceration, infection or atrophy of skin if injection site not rotated • More expensive • Client anxiety • Risks involved with sharps usage	Single- or multi-use vial of a drug or pre-filled syringe
Intravenous (IV) **injection**	• Very rapid and assured absorption therefore effective in critical care • Enables combined drug usage • Effective when unable to use oral routes	• Increased risks of side effects due to rapid absorption • Client anxiety and discomfort • Requires patent IV access via a cannula or central line • Increased risk of introducing infection • Risks involved with sharps usage • Can only be administered by an advanced nurse practitioner or doctor • Much less time to rectify adverse reactions	Single- or multi-use glass or plastic vial or pre-mixed infusion
Topical (Top)	• Painless • Inexpensive • Easy to use • Low risk of side effects • Local effect	• Cannot be used on broken skin • Difficult to use if client has reduced mobility • May stain skin or soil clothing	Cream Gel Paste

continued

Table 4.1 Advantages and disadvantages of different routes   cont'd

Route	Advantages	Disadvantages	Form(s)
Mucous membranes which include:	• Effective if client unable to use oral route • Rapid absorption due to systemic blood supply • Direct application to source, e.g. infection	• Risk of side effects • Client anxiety • Embarrassment and discomfort • Some routes cannot be used following surgery • Must have functional GI tract for rectal drugs	
sublingual (see Oral) **buccal**			Tablet Capsule
eyes			Cream Drops
ears (Aural) **nose** (Nasal)		• Underlying complications prevent use, e.g. ruptured eardrum	Drops Spray
vagina (PV)			Cream Pessary
rectum (PR)			Suppository Cream Enema
Inhalation i.e. Inhalers (Inh) and nebulizers (Neb)	• Rapid effect for relief of some respiratory symptoms • Sometimes used prophylactically pre-surgery	• Some side effects including sore mouth and throat (this can be reduced by using spacer device) • Client anxiety • Difficult to use with elderly or children • Support and teaching required for inhaler use • Expensive nebulizer equipment if used in chronic illness at home	Single-use plastic nebule or multidose inhaler (differing types)

Administering medicines to children

As most children find it difficult to swallow tablets, suspensions are usually prescribed. These are normally administered by using an oral syringe directly into the side of the child's mouth whilst their head is slightly tilted. However, some children prefer to use a medicine spoon; it is therefore always best to check with them before dispensing the medicine. The required volume should be calculated as follows:

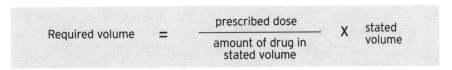

$$\text{Required volume} = \frac{\text{prescribed dose}}{\text{amount of drug in stated volume}} \times \text{stated volume}$$

For example:

You require 250 mg of a drug and you have a bottle with 500 mg of the drug in every 5 ml of liquid

$$\text{Required volume} = 250 \times \frac{5}{500} = 2.5\text{ml}$$

The child therefore requires 2.5 ml of liquid.

Drug errors

The Nursing and Midwifery Council (NMC 2002) encourages an open culture in relation to reporting drug errors. When investigating allegations of misconduct related to such errors the Council take great care to identify contextual issues, such as whether the error occurred due to incompetence; whether there was immediate disclosure in the client's best interests or, conversely, whether it was in some way concealed; or, indeed, whether the error may have resulted from some external cause, such as work pressures.

The NMC therefore urges ward managers to review each case individually and to consider the following:

- the type of drug involved
- the effect on the client
- whether the incident was disclosed and the timeframe involved
- hospital policies
- NMC guidelines
- the environment of care
- any other possible influencing factors
- the nurse(s)'s experience and whether they have been involved in any previous incidents.

In acting in the best interests of clients the procedure given below is recommended in the event of a drug error.

Procedure	Rationale
Inform the following people **immediately**: medical staff ward manager pharmacist client and their relatives if necessary	To alert medical and pharmaceutical staff to the error and request immediate review of client's condition. Ward manager informed to assess nursing practice and review possible cause for error. To maintain trust and confidence

Procedure	Rationale
Undertake any treatment or intervention prescribed by medical/pharmaceutical staff	To reduce risk of further complications and/or to counteract the error
Complete an untoward incident form	To identify risk and report to appropriate personnel. To record personal account of incident for further investigations by ward manager
Document the incident in client's records	Legal requirement to safeguard client and maintain communications through effective documentation
Monitor the client's condition and report any alteration in condition	To maintain client safety and well-being

Responding in the event of a fire

Fires within health care settings pose a major threat to all occupants in the building, clients obviously being the most vulnerable; fire safety strategies are therefore primarily based on the avoidance of fires.

Annual attendance at fire lectures is mandatory for all health care personnel to ensure that all staff are aware of their responsibilities in a fire situation and are conversant with how to reduce the risks of a fire occurring. Fire Safety Advisers are employed within all hospitals and most other health care settings, their role being to ensure that legislation is updated and applied to and within the workplace.

Whilst strategies may differ slightly for each health care setting due to, for example, building structure and numbers of staff, key principles underpinning the actions to be taken in the event of a fire and to reduce the potential for fire are based on the following legislation.

- The National Health Service and Community Care Act (1990)
- The Fire Precautions Act (1971) (amended by the Fire Safety and Safety at Places of Sport Act 1987)
- The Health and Safety at Work Act (1974)
- The Buildings Regulations Act (1991)

The basic principles are as follows:

- to ensure if at all possible that fires do not occur
- to ensure that fires are discovered rapidly, alarms are used and the fire brigade contacted immediately

- to ensure that the fire is extinguished quickly
- basic fire-fighting practice should be attempted only by staff that have been trained and only if it is considered safe to do so
- to provide safe means of escape or avoidance for everyone in all areas
- the spread of the fire is contained and delayed by structural and other means for as long as possible
- rehearsed evacuation routines are undertaken quickly
- evacuated areas are checked for the presence of clients and others and that a roll call is completed.

(Adapted from Department of Health and NHS Estates 1994.)

The general action points based on government and local policy to maintain fire safety within a health care setting are given below.

Action point	Rationale
Attend annual fire lecture	To ensure understanding of current fire procedures and policy
Observe no-smoking policies	To reduce the risk of fire from discarded cigarette
Observe parking restrictions within ground of workplace	To ensure easy access for emergency services
Identify all escape routes from the working area and ensure that these routes remain clear at all times	To allow efficient and effective management of evacuation
Ensure understanding of positioning and identification of all fire-fighting equipment within working area	To ensure efficient and effective use of all equipment as necessary
Ensure that fire doors are not wedged open	To ensure containment of fire
Do not use lifts to evacuate if fire present or fire alarm sounding	To ensure safety; reducing risk of smoke inhalation from lift shaft vacuum or risk of becoming trapped
Electrical equipment Ensure annual testing of all electrical equipment and report any defective piece of equipment for immediate repair. Reporting to manufacturer or in-house repairs department	To assess for faults thus reducing risk

Action point	Rationale
Switch off non-essential equipment when not in use	Potential fire hazards
Do not leave televisions on stand-by	Potential fire hazard
Client's own electrical equipment or adapters must be tested by in-house department prior to use	To ensure safety of all equipment
If safe to do so electrical equipment must be switched off at the wall socket if source of fire	**Ensuring personal safety first** - this action could slow down or stop the development of a fire
Gas Report any smell of gas immediately via emergency switchboard	To ensure immediate response and assistance
Do not switch on or off any item of electrical equipment	To reduce risk of fume ignition
Evacuate clients and staff	To ensure safety and evacuation from risk of inhalation or explosion
Ventilate area if possible and safe to do so	To reduce risk of inhalation and reduce concentration of gas collection

Fire extinguishers

Training is required for the use of fire extinguishers within the health care setting and this occurs at mandatory training sessions. Staff are advised to tackle fires only if they feel safe and happy to do so; containment, that is, closing a door on the fire, or evacuation are otherwise strongly advised.

Current European legislation means that the colour of fire extinguishers within health care settings is changing to reduce confusion and bring the UK in line with the rest of Europe. This is a gradual change as equipment is replaced following annual testing.

The fire extinguishers and equipment found commonly within health care settings are given in Table 4.2.

The key issues involved with responding in the event of a fire are:

- knowing the procedure for your working environment
- how to contact the emergency services
- who to call in an emergency

Table 4.2 Fire extinguishers and equipment

Type and colour	Type of fire	How it works	How to use
Foam Red with cream panel (New), cream (Old)	Wood, paper, linen, fabric, furnishing, liquid, oils, paints, solvents **NOT ELECTRICAL FIRES**	Cools Forms a film on liquid surface	Direct foam at base of fire, working across area. If fire vertical aim at top and work down. If liquid aim at outer edge and work around: do not aim directly onto liquid – this causes spread
Carbon dioxide Red with a black panel (New), black (Old)	Live electrical equipment	Displaces oxygen required to maintain combustion	**Switch off at mains if safe to do so.** Aim carbon dioxide in and around vents of electrical equipment
Fire blanket	Small fire, e.g. clothing, cooking, pans, oils or liquids	Smothers the fire thus reducing oxygen required for combustion	Place blanket over fire, protecting face and hands. **Turn off energy source if safe to do so.**

- when to evacuate and how to evacuate everyone safely from the area
- where exit and avoidance areas are situated
- what practical fire-fighting steps you can perform safely.

If we ensure that we understand all of the above we can act efficiently and effectively in maintaining the safety of clients, visitors, staff and ourselves.

Assessing an individual's ability to maintain a safe environment

Remember that assessment of an individual's ability to maintain a safe environment is only part of a holistic nursing assessment and should not be undertaken in isolation without reference to or consideration of the client's other activities of living.

Specific points to consider when assessing an individual's ability to maintain a safe environment include:

- *Physical*
  Degree of mobility
  Level of consciousness
  Level of aggression

- *Psychological*
  Knowledge of condition
  Depression
  Risk of self-harm
  Confusion
  Stress
  Anxiety
  Irritability
  Anger

- *Sociocultural*
  Health beliefs and values
  Level of family support
  Support from external agencies
  Hobbies/pastimes

- *Environmental*
  Client awareness of safety issues
  Spillages
  Confidentiality
  Communication systems
  Type of accommodation
  Ability to negotiate stairs
  Type of employment

- *Politico-economic*
  Limited finances/dependants
  Living conditions
  Employed/unemployed

Tips for child safety

- Lock away all household cleaners and medicines.
- Always keep pet food and water out of reach.
- When travelling by car always secure your children with a seat belt, safety seat or harness.
- Never leave a hot stove or barbecue unattended.

- Always bolt bookshelves to the wall.
- Keep some ipecacuanha syrup in the home to induce vomiting in poisoning.
- Limit exposure to the sun.
- Be sure they know what to do in the event of fire or other emergency.
- Check the recommended age limits for toys.
- Use safety gates on stairways.
- Install covers over unused electrical sockets and do not leave plugged-in appliances such as irons unattended.

References and further reading

Personal safety

Clough J (1998) Assessing and controlling risk. Nursing Standard 12(31): 49–54.
Home Office Communications Directorate (1996) Your Practical Guide to Crime Prevention. London: Home Office Communication Directorate.
http://www.nacab.org.uk
http://www.crimestoppers-uk.org
http://safer-community.net
The Suzy Lamplugh Trust (2002) Training and Resources. PO Box 17818, London SW14. http://www.suzylamplugh.org

Principles of health and safety at work

Brewer S (2001) Safe and sound... the Health and Safety at Work Act. Nursing Standard 15(34): 61.
Clough J (1998a) Rcn Continuing Education: Assessing and controlling risk. Nursing Standard 12(31): 49–54.
Clough J (1998b) Assessing and controlling risk. Emergency Nurse 6(3): 33–9.
Dimond B (2002) Enforcement of statutory duties for health and safety at work. British Journal of Nursing 11(11): 745–7.
EPIC (2001) The National Evidence-based Guidelines for Preventing Health-care Associated Infections. http://www.epic.tvu.ac.uk/epicphase/epic1.html (accessed 27 June 2003).
Girvin A, Girvin J (1998) Safe in your hands? Elderly Care 10(1): 36–7.
Health and Safety Executive (1999a) Health and Safety Law – What you should Know. http://www.open.gov.uk/hse/hsehome.htm (accessed 18 February 2003).
Health and Safety Executive (1999b) Ionising Radiation – Radiation Protection. http://www.open.gov.uk/hse/hsehome.htm (accessed 18 February 2003).
Health and Safety Executive (1999c) COSHH Regulations – COSHH in a Hurry. http://www.open.gov.uk/hse/hsehome.htm.
National Audit Office (1996) Health & Safety in NHS Acute Hospital Trusts in England. London: The Stationery Office.
Parker LJ (1999) Managing and maintaining a safe environment in the hospital setting. British Journal of Nursing 8(16): 1053–8.
Ransom E (1999) Health and safety work equipment – is it harmful to health? Synergy April: 18–19.
Rogers R, Salvage J, Cowell R (1999) Nurses at Risk – A Guide to Health and Safety at Work, 2nd edn. London: Macmillan Press.

Universal precautions

Ayliffe GAJ, Babb JR, Taylor LJ (2000) Hospital Acquired Infection – Principles and Prevention, 3rd edn. Oxford: Butterworth & Heinemann.

Ayliffe GAJ, Fraise AP, Geddes AM, Mitchell K (2000) Control of Hospital Infection – A Practical Handbook, 4th edn. London: Arnold Publishers.

Begany T (2000) Can handwashing increase the risk of transmitting infections? Respiratory Reviews 5(8): 12–14.

Buchanan J (2001) Using research to improve infection control practice. Professional Nurse 16(5): 1091–4.

Department of Health (2001) Standard Principles for Preventing Hospital-Acquired Infections. London: Department of Health.

Department of Health (2002) Getting Ahead of The Curve – A Strategy for Combating Infectious Diseases (including other aspects of health protection). London: Department of Health.

Kerr J (1998) Handwashing. Nursing Standard 12(51): 35–39, 41–42.

Mandal KB, Wilkins EGL, Dunbar EM, Mayon-White RT (1996) Infectious Diseases – Lecture Notes, 5th edn. London: Blackwell Sciences.

May D (2001) Infection control. Nursing Standard 14(28): 51–7.

National Audit Office Press Notice (2000) The Management and Control of Hospital Acquired Infection In Acute NHS Trusts in England. http://www.nao.gov.uk/pn/9900230.htm (accessed 19 February 2003).

NHS (2000) Decontamination of Medical Devices – HSC (2000)032. London: Department of Health.

NHS (1995) Hospital Laundry Arrangements for Used and Infected Linen – Health Service Circular (95)18. London: Department of Health.

Norton L (2000) Testing gloves used for common nursing tasks. Professional Nurse 15(6): 377–80.

Parker J (1999) Importance of handwashing in the prevention of cross-infection. British Journal of Nursing 8(11): 716–19.

Plowman R, Graves N, Taylor L, et al. (1999) Socio-economic Burden of Hospital Acquired Infections. London: Department of Health.

Royal College of Nursing (2001a) Good Practice in Infection Control – Guidance for Nurses Working in General Practice. London: Royal College of Nursing.

Royal College of Nursing (2001b) Be Sharp – Be Safe. London: Royal College of Nursing.

Stone SP (1998) The effect of an enhanced infection control policy on the incidence of Clostridium difficile and Methicillin Resistant Staphylococcus aureus colonisation in acute elderly medical clients. Age and Ageing 27: 561–8.

Ward D (2000) Handwashing facilities in the clinical area: a literature review. British Journal of Nursing 9(2): 82–6.

White C (2002) UK has worst MRSA rates. Nursing Times 98(12): 8.

Monitoring pulse

Evans D, Hodgkinson B, Berry J (1999) Vital Signs. A Systematic Review, No 4. Adelaide: The Joanna Briggs Institute for Evidence Based Nursing and Midwifery, Royal Adelaide Hospital.

McConnell E (1993) Assessing pulse deficit. Nursing 23(11): 18.

Nichol M, Bavin C, Bedford-Turner S, et al. (2000) Essential Nursing Skills. Edinburgh: Harcourt.

Torrance C, Elley K (1997a) Assessing pulse: Part 1 Practical procedures for nurses supplement. Nursing Times 93(41): 1–2.

Torrance C, Elley K (1997b) Assessing pulse: Part 2 Practical procedures for nurses supplement. Nursing Times 93(42): 1–2.

Monitoring blood pressure

Ballie L (Ed) (2001) Developing Practical Skills. London: Arnold.
British Hypertension Society (1999) Blood Pressure Measurement CD ROM. London: British Medical Association Publishing.
Edwards S (1997) Recording blood pressure. Professional Nurse 13(2 suppl): 8-10.
Feather C (2001) Equipment for blood pressure measurement. Professional Nurse 16(11): 1458-62.
O'Brien E, Davison M (1994) Blood pressure measurement: rational and ritual actions. British Journal of Nursing 3(8): 393-6.
Smith GR (2000) Devices for blood pressure measurement. Professional Nurse 15(5): 337-40.
Toms E (1995) Vital observations. Nursing Times 89(51): 32-4. (Also try http://w3.abdn.ac.uk/BHS for a video of the procedure.)

Principles of asepsis

Anon (1996) Proposed recommended practices for establishing and maintaining a sterile field. AORN Journal 63(1): 211-17.
Barber LA (2002) Clean technique or sterile technique? Let's take a moment to think. Journal of Wocn 29(1): 29-32.
Briggs S, Jones V (1996) The principles of aseptic technique in wound care. Professional Nurse 11(12): 805-808.
Gilmour D (1999) Redefining aseptic technique. Journal of Community Nursing 13(7): 22-6.
Gray M (2001) Clean versus sterile technique when changing wound dressings. Journal of Wocn 28(3): 125-8.
Hollinworth H (1998) Using a non-sterile technique in wound care. Professional Nurse 13(4): 226-9.
Rowley S (2001) Aseptic non-touch technique. Nursing Times 97(7): VI-VIII.
Trevelyan J (1996) Wound cleansing: principles and practice. Nursing Times 92(16): 46-7.
Xavier G (1999) Asepsis. Nursing Standard 13(36): 49-53.

Responding in the event of a cardiac arrest

American Heart Association in collaboration with the International Committee on Resuscitation (ILCOR) (2000) Guidelines 2000 for Cardiopulmonary Resuscitation and Emergency Cardiovascular Care. An international consensus on science. Resuscitation 46: 29-71.
ARTO (1993) Standards in Resuscitation Training for Hospital Staff. Association of Resuscitation Training Officers. www.arto.info (accessed 27 June 2003).
British Medical Association and Royal College of Nursing (1999) Decisions relating to Cardiopulmonary Resuscitation. A joint statement from the British Medical Association, Resuscitation Council (UK) and Royal College of Nursing. London: British Medical Association.
International Liaison Committee on Resuscitation (1997) An advisory statement by the Basic Life Support Working Group of the International Liaison Committee on Resuscitation 34: 101-107. Dallas: American Heart Association.
Mackway-Jones K, Molyneux E, Phillips B, Wieteska S (2001) Advanced Paediatric Life Support: The Practical Approach, 3rd edn. London: BMJ Books.
NHS Executive (1997) Service Standards for Emergency Medical Admissions. London: NHS Executive.
Royal College of Physicians (1987) Resuscitation from Cardiopulmonary Arrest: Training and Organisation: A Report of the Royal College of Physicians. London: Royal College of Physicians.

Resuscitation Council UK (2000a) Basic Life Support Resuscitation Guidelines 2000. http://www.resus.org.uk (accessed 26 June 2003).

Resuscitation Council UK (2000b) Paediatric Basic Life Support Resuscitation Guidelines 2000. http://www.resus.org.uk (accessed 26 June 2003).

UKRC (1996) Should Relatives Witness Resuscitation? A Report from a Project Team of the Resuscitation Council. London: Resuscitation Council UK.

Administration of medicines

Downie G, Mackenzie J, Williams A (1999) Pharmacology and Drug Management for Nurses, 2nd edn. London: Churchill Livingstone.

Haigh S (2002) How to calculate drug dosage accurately: advice for nurses. Professional Nurse 18(1): 54-7.

Henry JA (2001) New Guide to Medicines and Drugs. London: British Medical Association.

British Medical Association (2003) Nurse Prescribers' Formulary. London: British Medical Association.

Nursing and Midwifery Council (2002a) Guidelines for the administration of medicines. London: Nursing and Midwifery Council (or http://www.nmc-uk.org or publications@nmc-uk.org) (accessed 26 June 2003).

Nursing and Midwifery Council (2002b) Code of Professional Conduct. London: Nursing and Midwifery Council (or http://www.nmc-uk.org or publications@nmc-uk.org).

Rodger MA, King L (2000) Drawing up and administering intramuscular injections: a review of the literature. Journal of Advanced Nursing 31(3): 574.

Workman B (1999) Safe injection techniques. Nursing Standard 13(9): 47-53.

Zuckerman J (2000) The importance of injecting vaccines into muscle: Different clients need different needle sizes. British Medical Journal 321(7271): 1237-8.

Responding in the event of a fire

Department of Health, NHS Estates (1994) Firecode – Policy and Principles. London: HMSO.

BSEN 3 (1996) Portable Fire Extinguishers.

BS7863 (1996) Recommendations for colour coding to indicate the extinguishing media contained in portable fire extinguishers.

www.bsi-global.com (British Standards Institution).

Assessing an individual's ability to maintain a safe environment

Hogson R, Simpson PM (1999) Foundations of Nursing Practice. London: Macmillan Press.

Roper N, Logan WW, Tierney A (1996) The Elements of Nursing. Edinburgh: Churchill Livingstone.

Walsh M (2002) Watson's Clinical Nursing and Related Sciences, 6th edn. London: Ballière Tindall.

Chapter 5

Eating and drinking

Catherine Waskett

Introduction

Good nutritional status is essential to an individual's health and well-being. Many clients have an increased need for nutrients because of the extra demands being placed on the body by illness. Poor nutritional status has been associated with delayed recovery and an increase in mortality, which also increase the cost of providing health care. In addition, adequate nutrition not only promotes growth and repair of tissues but also aids recovery from surgery, disease and trauma.

Unfortunately recent reports have highlighted that many people in hospital are malnourished on admission but also that they often receive inadequate nutrition once in our care. In an attempt to address this problem, 'Food and Nutrition' has been included in the first wave of 'Essence of Care' documents produced by the Department of Health. These documents outline benchmarks for good practice with the aim of improving the quality of care. In relation to food and nutrition 10 outcomes have been identified (see Table 5.1). It is important that nurses and other health care professionals recognize the importance of their role in the prevention of malnutrition, and be able to identify clients at risk and plan appropriate interventions.

The factors that may affect eating and drinking include:

- *physical* arising from alteration in the structure, function or processes of the gastro-intestinal tract and associated systems, for example ulcerative colitis, diabetes mellitus, facial disfigurement
- *psychological* such as depression, anxiety and anorexia
- *sociocultural*, for example vegetarians, vegan or religious persuasion
- *environmental* including unpleasant smells, inaccessibility of shops
- *politico-economic*, for example lack of finances.

This chapter outlines the common terminology associated with eating and drinking and some of the principles and practices when assessing and meeting the nutritional needs of the client. These include assessing an individual's nutritional and hydration status; assisting clients in selecting

Table 5.1 Benchmarks for practice

Factor	Benchmark for practice
1 Screening and assessment to identify client's nutritional needs	All clients should be assessed on admission and clients deemed 'at risk' should undergo further assessment
2 Care should be planned, implemented and evaluated for all clients requiring further nutritional assessment	Plans of care should be readily available and ongoing, demonstrating evaluation and reassessment of care needs
3 A conducive environment	An environment conducive to eating and drinking should be provided
4 Assistance to eat and drink	Clients should receive any care and assistance they require with eating and drinking
5 Obtaining food	Clients should have sufficient information to enable them to obtain the food and drink they require
6 Food provided	Food provided should meet the needs of the client
7 Food availability	Meal times should be set but clients should be offered a replacement meal if they miss the set timed meal, and snacks should be readily available at any time
8 Food presentation	Food should be presented to clients in an appealing manner
9 Monitoring nutrition	The amount of food and drink a client actually takes in should be monitored and recorded, and should lead to action if there is cause for concern
10 Eating to promote health	Every opportunity should be taken to educate clients about the importance of nutrition in promoting their own health

Source: Department of Health (2001)

appropriate meals/fluids; monitoring nutritional and fluid intake; assisting clients with eating and drinking; feeding dependent clients and clients with potential swallowing difficulties; and providing first aid to a client who is choking. The chapter concludes with references and further reading.

Common terminology

Anorexia	Lack of appetite
Anorexia nervosa	A psychiatric disorder characterized by intense fear of becoming overweight, even when emaciated
Anosmia	The loss of sense of smell
Appetite	The psychological stimulus to eat that may be connected with and triggered by emotional stimuli
Asphyxia	Suffocation. Occurs when the tissues are unable to obtain adequate amounts of oxygen
Basal metabolic rate	The amount of energy needed by the body for essential processes when at complete rest but awake
Body mass index	A figure derived from a person's height and weight that indicates whether that weight is acceptable
Bulimia nervosa	An eating disorder in which binge eating is followed by depression and guilt, self-induced vomiting and purging
Dysphagia	Painful or difficult swallowing; may result from local mouth or throat disorders, anxiety, or certain central nervous system disorders
Halitosis	Bad breath
Malabsorption	Inadequate or disordered absorption of nutrients from the intestinal canal
Malnutrition	The state of being poorly nourished. May be caused by inadequate food or deficiency of some essential nutrients, or by malabsorption due to a metabolic defect that prevents the body from utilizing nutrients properly
Nutrition	The science related to the food requirements of the body
PEG (Percutaneous Endoscopic Gastronomy)	A tube inserted into the stomach through the abdominal wall to feed clients. May be temporary or permanent.
Turgor	Resistance of the skin to deformation when pinched. Related mainly to age, but can be a sign of dehydration.

Assessing an individual's nutritional status

Nurses are in an ideal position to assess a client's nutritional status, and thus identify if they are at risk from malnutrition. It should include taking a nutritional history, including consideration of the factors identified below that can interfere with nutritional status, along with physical measurements (see Figure 5.1). There are also local and national nutritional assessment tools; however, not all of them are research based. Most of them consist of a list of questions with the answers being scored (see Figure 5.2). The total score gives an indication of the client's nutritional status and susceptibility to malnutrition. If a tool is not being used, the client on admission should at least be asked the following questions:

1 Have you been eating more or less than usual?
2 Have you unintentionally lost or gained weight?
3 How tall are you?
4 What is your normal weight?

The weight of a client on admission can act as a baseline and if there is cause for concern then weekly weight measurements should be taken. A greater than 10 per cent loss in body weight in less than three months indicates that the client is malnourished and needs to be referred to the

Figure 5.1 Are you the right weight for your height?

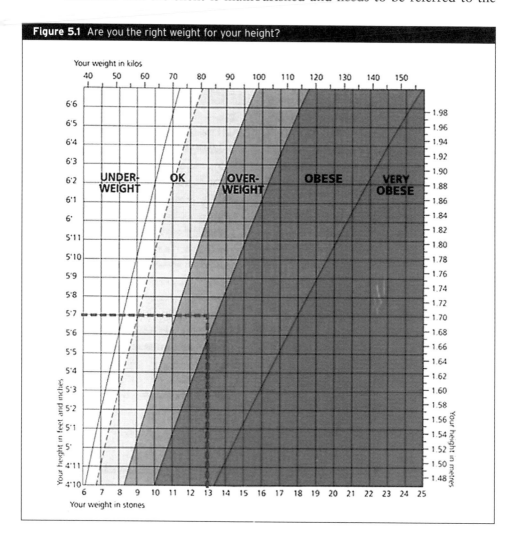

dietician. It is also important to remember that clients who are obese can equally be malnourished, as they may not be ingesting an adequate range of nutrients.

Figure 5.2 Example of nutrition risk assessment tool	Adapted from BAPEN (1996)

	Score
Weight loss, unintentional in past three months	
• No weight loss	0
• 0-3 kg weight loss	1
• 3-6 kg weight loss	2
• > 6 kg weight loss	3
BMI	
• 20 or more	0
• 18-19	1
• 15-17	2
• < 15	3
Appetite	
• Good, manages most of three meals/day	0
• Poor, leaves percentage of meals provided	2
• Nil, unable to eat	3
Ability to eat/retain food	
• No difficulties eating, independent. No diarrhoea/vomiting	0
• Problems handling food. Occasional diarrhoea/vomiting	1
• Difficulties swallowing. Needs modified consistency. Moderate diarrhoea/vomiting	2
• Unable to take food orally. Unable to swallow. Severe diarrhoea/vomiting/ malabsorption	3
Total score	

Score	Action
0-3 low risk	No action required, weigh weekly
4-5 needs monitoring	Encourage eating and drinking. Possibly food record charts. Repeat score after one week
6-12 high risk	Refer to dietician

Remember that assessment of the activity of eating and drinking is only part of a holistic nursing assessment and should not be undertaken in isolation without reference to or consideration of the client's other activities of living.

Specific points to consider when assessing individuals' nutritional and hydration status include:

- *Physical*

  What is the condition of the mouth, teeth and gums? Poor oral hygiene, a sore mouth or ill-fitting dentures can cause difficulty when eating.

  Does the client have halitosis? This may indicate poor oral hygiene or dehydration.

  Appearance: dry, scaly skin may indicate that the client is malnourished or dehydrated.

  Does the client have sunken eye sockets? This may be suggestive of dehydration.

  Is their hair dull, lifeless or in bad condition? This can be an indication of poor nutritional status.

  Is their clothing loose or tight, or rings or dentures slack, indicating a recent weight gain or loss?

  Does the client have limited hand dexterity resulting in difficulty in manipulating cutlery (for example rheumatoid arthritis)?

  Does the client have any visual deficits, physical handicap or positional difficulty? These may interfere with independence in eating and drinking.

  Are they nauseous or vomiting? Symptoms such as these will prevent clients from eating, even if they feel hungry. Do they have any food allergies?

  Are they able to chew and swallow? Certain conditions, such as motor neurone disease, stroke and cerebral palsy, can cause problems with chewing and swallowing and leave the patient at risk of aspiration and/or malnutrition.

  Any diarrhoea or constipation? This can lead to malabsorption syndrome.

  Does the client require starving prior to surgery/investigations or because of condition? For example, intestinal obstruction carries a high risk of malnutrition.

  Any pain, stress, fatigue or reduced physical activity? This often accompanies illness and can result in a loss of appetite.

  Is the client receiving any medications that can adversely affect their appetite?

  Is the physical effort of eating too great for the client? This can be true for people with heart failure or emphysema, or children with congenital heart disease.

Has the client any additional nutritional requirements due to wound or bone healing or loss, for example dehydration following burn injury?

Does the client have any pressure sores? These are often associated with poor nutrition.

Is there any deterioration in a client's level of consciousness or mental state (for example confusion) that may affect their ability and desire to eat or drink?

Does the client require any special diet that may restrict their choice, for example renal disease, diabetes mellitus, malabsorption syndromes, obesity?

Does the client have a learning difficulty affecting their ability to select an appropriate diet or prepare food?

Remember that children have higher metabolic rates than adults, and so require more energy. They also need to eat the correct amount and type of food to support growth in adulthood.

- *Psychological*

    Is the client depressed or bereaved, thereby affecting appetite and motivation to prepare food?

    Is the client turning to food as a source of comfort, resulting in over-eating during periods of loneliness, insecurity or depression?

    Is the client suffering from paranoia and not eating because of fear of being poisoned?

    Is the client suffering from stress or anxiety, which is suppressing their appetite?

    Does the client have any deviations in eating patterns, for example anorexia nervosa or bulimia nervosa?

    Does the individual neglect their diet as a result of a busy, stressful life?

- *Sociocultural*

    Are there any cultural factors (that is, the collection of attitudes, taboos and beliefs) influencing the individual's diet and eating habits? For example, some people may feel that without a daily hot meal their diet is incomplete.

    Any other food ideologies that might influence the individual's motivation to alter their food habits?

    Are there any religious beliefs/customs influencing their diet and eating habits? (See Table 5.2 for guidance.)

    Is the client vegetarian or vegan?

    Are they following any fad diets?

    Do they have any spurious health beliefs resulting in them following a diet that is too restricted to meet their nutritional needs?

- *Environmental*

    Does the client have adequate food preparation and cooking equipment (or access to it)?

Do they have shops or supermarkets in the vicinity?

Are these conducive? Local shops may not have as good a choice as supermarkets and can be more expensive.

Is their appetite likely to be affected by the hospital environment, for example unpleasant/unfamiliar smells and sounds.

- *Politico-economic*

Is the client unemployed or on a low income? Elderly people or those with children may be living beneath the poverty line and low-income families are less likely than higher-income families to eat vegetables and fresh fruit.

Does the client rely on starchy 'filler' foods such as white bread, biscuits, cakes, sweets and fatty foods?

Is their vitamin and mineral status compromised as a result?

Does shopping for food involve a bus journey costing time and money?

Does the client lack knowledge about the importance of good nutrition?

Are they unable to buy suitable food or to prepare it?

Lack of knowledge may also lead to errors in making up bottle feeds for infants resulting in over-concentration that can cause harm, or conversely, weak feeds, resulting in failure to gain weight.

Table 5.2 Religious beliefs/customs influencing diet and eating habits

Religion	Special dietary needs
Buddhism	Although it does not appear in the teachings many Buddhists follow a vegetarian or vegan diet as Buddha commends a harmless life. Strict or ordained Buddhists may decline anything but a vegan diet and in addition may refuse food after midday (unless for medicinal purposes) as this acknowledges that people often indulge a craving for food by eating more than is needed. As they interfere with judgement the uses of intoxicants such as alcohol are likely to be resisted. Buddhists may also refuse sedatives, tranquillizers and opiates as these drugs can also have an impact on their consciousness and awareness
Christianity	There are an estimated seven million practising Christians in the UK and Christianity is found in many other countries around the world. Although the core beliefs remain the same, the interpretation of its teachings may be modified by local culture and custom. It is impossible to include the dietary customs of every branch of Christianity and therefore the less familiar branches of Christianity are highlighted. These are the Afro-Caribbean Christian community in the UK of which the main churches are Methodist, Anglican, Pentecostal and Church of God, and secondly Christian Orthodoxy of which the Greek Orthodox Church is an example. Afro-Caribbean Christians usually have no dietary restrictions although most of the community may not eat pork. Traditional foods include rice and peas, chicken, curried goat or mutton, yam and green bananas (plantains). Some hospitals provide Caribbean dishes for patients. Older people usually prefer traditional foods, which can cause problems when they are admitted to hospital. Traditionally, Christians are supposed to refrain from eating meat during Lent, a 40-day period before Easter, which begins on Ash Wednesday. Fish should be served instead. In Christian communities fish as an alternative to meat is also traditionally served on Fridays

cont'd

Table 5.2 Religious beliefs/customs influencing diet and eating habits   cont'd

Religion	Special dietary needs
Christianity (cont'd)	Within Christian Orthodoxy there are no dietary restrictions except during periods of fasting, which are seen as spiritual catharsis. Unlike Muslims, who abstain from food from dawn to dusk during holy periods, for Orthodox Christians fasting means abstaining from animal and dairy products.
	The Church requires healthy adults to fast at least three days before taking communion and during the holy periods of Easter (50 days up to Easter Sunday), the Assumption of the Virgin Mary (August 1-14) and Christmas (40 days up to Christmas day).
	In practice, apart from the older generation few people observe the extended fasting rules. Those wishing to take holy communion usually fast for three days during the year, apart from before Easter and Christmas. The sick and young children are excluded from fasting
Hinduism	Many Hindus restrict what they eat and drink on religious grounds and some may refuse food that has been prepared by other people as they cannot be sure that the cooking methods have adhered to the purity code of the religion. They may also avoid processed foods or any food containing animal products.
	Vegetarianism is regarded highly as an indication of spirituality, therefore a strict Hindu vegetarian who eats any food containing meat, fish or egg products is likely to feel spiritually polluted. The cow is a sacred animal that is generally protected and revered but the pig is perceived as a scavenging animal whose meat is dirty so Hindus will not eat beef or pork. Some Hindus may fast on certain occasions as they believe it has spiritual benefits. In addition, close relatives, especially women, often fast and say special prayers for the recovery of someone ill. Some may fast in thanksgiving for a successful operation or recovery
Islam (Muslim)	Permissible food is referred to as halal. Non-permissible food is called haram. Halal foods include halal meat, fish, fresh fruit and vegetables, milk, eggs and cheese. Halal meat comes from an animal that has been slaughtered during a prayer ritual.
	Haram foods include pork, non-halal meat, gelatine products and alcoholic drinks. Care must be taken when serving food to ensure that halal food does not become contaminated with haram food. Muslims also eat with their right hand and consider it rude to be handed anything in the left hand, especially a glass of water, as the left hand is used for washing the genital area.
	During the month of Ramadan Muslims are only allowed to eat at certain times of the day. People eat and drink before sunrise and sunset and then signify their intention to keep the fast by rinsing their mouth with water. No food or drink is consumed during daylight hours. The fast is broken at sunset usually by eating a piece of fruit or a date, followed by a main meal. Children are expected to start praying and observing the fast when they reach puberty. Muslims who are ill are exempt from fasting, but some still fast and may also omit or refuse medication. To accommodate fasting the times that medicines are due may be rescheduled or the dose possibly changed.
	The use of tobacco, alcohol and other intoxicating substances is prohibited
Judaism	Jewish people are required to eat kosher food, which is food that is fit to be eaten in accordance with Jewish law. There are lots of laws relating to kosher food so it is always advisable to ask patients or their families what their custom is.
	Broadly speaking the laws on food govern two areas – food types that cannot be eaten, such as pork and shellfish and their derivatives, and the utensils in which food must be cooked. Milk and meat cannot be eaten or cooked together. Therefore orthodox households always have two sets of pots and pans, cutlery and crockery – one for dairy products and one for meat dishes. Hospital cutlery and plates cannot be used.
	These laws are usually followed by orthodox Jews, but not by all. As the cooking methods as well as food types are different, offering a patient a vegetarian meal is not a

Table 5.2 Religious beliefs/customs influencing diet and eating habits

Religion	Special dietary needs
Judaism (cont'd)	suitable alternative. Hospitals can order kosher meals, which can be reheated in the hospital ovens. The meals also come supplied with plates and cutlery. Orthodox Jews wait up to six hours between eating meat and dairy products and some drink only kosher milk. All medication is permitted except when there is an alternative
Mormon (Church of Jesus Christ of the Latter Day Saints)	No particular dietary laws or customs
Rastafarian	Many Rastafarians follow a system of hygiene and dietary laws that uphold and advocate a naturalistic and holistic lifestyle. The body is regarded as the temple of god, which should be protected from contamination. Food is considered to have a key influence on the well-being of body and soul. What is acceptable is down to individual choice but natural food that is as pure and fresh as possible (known as ital) is highly valued. Pork, predatory fish and some types of crustaceans are regarded as especially unwholesome. Dairy products, sweets, sugar-based beverages, white flour, preserved foods (those in tins or containing additives) and anything containing salt is generally avoided. Alcohol is rarely taken. The most orthodox Rastafarians are vegans
Sikhism	Dietary customs vary from not eating beef, fish or eggs to vegetarianism. Ritualistic fasting is forbidden by the faith but may be performed as part of a patient's culture, especially by Sikhs whose families originated in or near Hindu towns or villages. Eating meat prepared as part of a ritual, for example halal meat, is forbidden. Many Sikhs also avoid veal and beef out of respect for the Hindu faith, in which the cow is a sacred animal. Ensuring that an accurate description is available of the ingredients in hospital food may reassure Sikh patients, particularly older people who may refuse food they do not recognize

Calculating body mass index

The answers to the questions about the client's height and weight are needed to calculate the body mass index (BMI) (see Figure 5.2). The BMI is determined by considering a client's weight in relation to height, and is a better indication of healthy ranges for body weight than weight alone. N.B. This calculation is unsuitable for use with babies, children, pregnant women, and amputees. In addition if an individual has a large amount of muscle mass he may be incorrectly identified as 'obese' on the BMI range.

To calculate the BMI the following formula is used:

$$\text{BMI calculation} = \frac{\text{weight (kg)}}{\text{height}^2 \text{ (m)}}$$

For example:
If a female client's weight is 50 kg and height is 1.68 m the BMI is:

$$\frac{50}{1.68 \times 1.68} \ = \ 17.7$$

Reference ranges for a desirable BMI are:

- men: 20.5-25.0
- women: 19-24
- 25-30 = overweight
- above 30 = obese

The example above of 17.7 indicates that the client is underweight and therefore malnourished.

Whilst generally less accurate, Figure 5.1 offers an 'at a glance chart' to help determine the height/weight ratio.

Assessing an individual's hydration status

The importance of water

At least 70 per cent of the body is composed of water. The body's cells rely on having the correct amount of water in order to work efficiently. Water provides the main transport system of the body and is the basic component of extracellular fluid, lymph, blood and urine, the main 'transporters'. Body cells become selectively permeable during the movement of dissolved substances (solutes) across the cell membrane. This ensures that, in health, the concentration of water in the cell is maintained at a constant level enabling the cells to work efficiently. In this way the whole body is maintained 'in balance' and the person is well (homeostasis).

Water forms three distinct compartments within the body:

1 intracellular (cellular) content (30 litres)
2 extracellular fluid content (12 litres)
3 vascular content (3 litres)

All of these compartments need a stable water content to work efficiently. If one of the compartments becomes low in water content, the body is dehydrated. In addition, the compartments become dehydrated in a specific order. The vascular system is always first, followed by the extracellular compartment and, lastly, the cellular compartment is affected.

Water is not only a transport system – it is also an excretory pathway. Water is always lost from the body, the majority as urine. Visible sweat from the skin, along with 'insensible' sweat (sweat taking place without us being aware of it), as well as the water vapour we breathe out accounts for approximately 2.5–3 litres of water loss daily in adults, which needs to be replaced (see Table 5.3). Note that these losses are increased after exercise, so extra water needs to be consumed.

Table 5.3 Bodily intake and output of water (adult)

Intake	ml	Output	ml
Water intake as fluid	1000	From lungs as water in expired air	500
Water intake as solid food	1200	From kidneys in urine	1500
Water produced in body cells as a by-product of metabolism	400	From skin in 'insensible' perspiration	450
		From gut in faeces	150
TOTAL	**2600**		**2600**

Signs and symptoms of dehydration

- The first symptom of dehydration is generally thirst.
- A dry and coated tongue is a strong indicator of dehydration. A client may find talking difficult due to the tongue sticking to the roof of the mouth.
- The client may have increased skin turgor and the skin can be dry and scaly in appearance.
- The eyes may appear shrunken into their sockets.
- An infant's fontanels may be sunken.
- The urine may be dark in colour and low in amount as the body tries to conserve water.
- A client's blood pressure is affected because the vascular compartment is the first to be affected by dehydration.
- A client's heartrate will begin to rise in an attempt to maintain blood pressure.
- Initially, however, the loss of water may raise blood pressure as a result of the blood-cell content being more concentrated, in effect 'thickening' the

blood and therefore needing a higher pressure to get this thicker blood through the vascular system. This can cause headaches.

- Eventually, however, if the client continues to lose fluid, the blood pressure will fall and if the losses are not replaced the client will develop hypovoleamic shock.
- Chronic dehydration (often due to people not wanting to or being unable to drink or take adequate fluids, if for example worried about urinary incontinence) can lead to renal problems and constipation.
- Conditions that can cause dehydration need to be identified and considered. Everyday causes of dehydration include:

  not drinking enough
  alcohol
  smoking
  caffeine
  sunstroke
  central heating
  infection and pyrexia
  diarrhoea and vomiting
  illness (e.g. diabetes mellitus).

In adults, drinking several pints of water can alleviate dehydration quickly. However, when the cause of the dehydration is infection or illness, further treatment, such as intravenous fluids, may be needed. Fluid replacement in infants and children must be undertaken with great care and be calculated exceptionally accurately given the much smaller volumes of fluid involved.

Assisting clients in selecting appropriate meals/fluids

To be able to assist clients in the selection of an appropriate diet it is important that health carer professionals understand the key components of a nutritious diet and are aware of factors affecting nutritional demands in the healthy individual. In addition, health promotion is a statutory requirement of the registered nurse so knowledge of what constitutes a healthy diet and fluid intake for the client is crucial. An in-depth discussion of what the constituents of a healthy balanced diet are is beyond the scope of this chapter and will require further reading, but an outline of the required nutrients and their role within the body is given in Table 5.4.

In addition to knowing about the various nutrients it is important to know what *foods* make up a balanced diet. This can be summarized by the percentages given below and is illustrated in Figure 5.3 (p. 144).

- Starchy foods: 33%
- Fruit and vegetables: 33%
- Milk and dairy products: 14%
- Meat and alternatives (e.g. tofu, pulses): 12%
- Oils, fats, fatty foods, sugars, sugary foods (and alcohol, if taken): 8%

Table 5.4 Nutrients and their role within the body

Nutrient	Function
Protein	• Used for building, growth or recovery of cells and tissues • Major constituent of hormones, enzymes and antibodies • Found in meat, fish, eggs, pulses (peas, beans and lentils), nuts, soya and textured vegetable protein (TVP)
Fats	• Source of energy • Component of cell membranes • Found in solid fats and liquid oils, in dairy produce and in hidden fat in food, for example between muscle fibres in meats, as oils, nuts, cereals, vegetables and fruit (especially avocados), or as fat used in the processing and cooking of foods
Carbohydrates	• Source of energy and fibre to aid digestion and bowel function and divided into starches and sugars • Starchy foods include bread, rice, cereals, pasta, potatoes, flour, crispbread, porridge and chapattis • Sugars are divided into intrinsic sugars (contained within plant cell walls) and extrinsic sugars (which are free in solution in the food, as in fruit juice, added sugar and honey in foods, and lactose in milk) • Processed foods, chocolates, sweets and snacks are dense sources of sugar
Vitamins	• Essential in small quantities for the normal growth and functioning of the body
Minerals	• Important building substances (e.g. calcium in bone tissues) and for the normal functioning of the body
Water	• Used for building, as a solvent for carrying nutrients and waste, and involved in temperature regulation
Fibre	• Dietary fibre is not strictly speaking a nutrient, but its presence in diet is necessary for the movement of food through the gastro-intestinal tract. It is divided into two types – soluble and insoluble – Soluble fibre is found in pulses, oats, barley, beans and lentils and also in fruit and vegetables – Insoluble fibre is found in wheat-based breakfast cereals, bread, rice, maize, pasta, fruits and vegetables. Bran hurries the food through, reducing the absorption of vitamins and minerals, producing a sort of scouring pad effect, and should be used with caution

Factors that influence a healthy individual's nutritional needs

- **Age**: Children have higher metabolic rates than adults, and so require more energy and also need to eat the correct amount and type of food to support growth. In adulthood, as age increases, energy requirements decrease due to the lower metabolic rate of older people compared with younger adults.
- **Sex**: Men require more energy, hence calories, because they have a higher metabolic rate than women due to their relatively greater muscle mass.
- **Amount of physical activity**: As energy is used as fuel, the higher the level of activity the more energy is used up and more calories are required.
- **Height and build**: The bigger the size of the body, the larger the amount of nutrients required to maintain cells.
- **Pregnancy**: The rapid growth of the foetus, during the second and third trimesters of pregnancy, changes nutritional needs although the exact changes vary from woman to woman. In particular, the demand for energy, protein and vitamins A, B, C and D are higher. However, 'eating for two' is not necessary as decreased maternal energy towards the end of pregnancy often compensates for the increased energy requirements of the foetus. In addition, the average British diet usually contains sufficient protein to meet the increased demands.
- **Lactation**: Women who are breast-feeding require more energy and therefore increased calorific intake (up to 500 calories a day) as well as increased vitamin A, C and D and calcium intake. Table 5.5 gives the estimated energy requirements for adults.

Table 5.5 Energy requirements for adults

Estimated average energy requirements for energy - men		Estimated average energy requirements for energy - women	
Age	**kcal**	**Age**	**kcal**
18-34		18-54	
• Sedentary	2500	• Most occupations	2100
• Moderately active	2800	• Very active	2500
• Very active	3350	55-74 (assuming sedentary)	1900
35-64			
• Sedentary	2400	75+ (assuming sedentary)	1680
• Moderately active	2750	Pregnancy	2400
• Very active	3300		
65-74 (assuming sedentary)	2400	Lactation	2750
75+ (assuming sedentary)	2150		

These healthy eating recommendations need to be considered, along with client choice, when assisting an individual to choose a healthy meal. It is good practice to spend time with the client to establish their likes and dislikes. If you are with the client you can direct their choice towards the correct food to choose. For example, if a client is underweight or has a wound or pressure sore, you can encourage them to choose high-protein/high-calorie options to help facilitate weight gain and provide them with sufficient amounts of protein, which is required for effective wound healing.

If a person's appetite is very poor or due to illness they have increased nutritional demands as a result of higher metabolic rate, food intake may be insufficient to meet nutritional needs. In these instances a wide range of supplements can be used. Supplements are used to increase the nutritional value of oral intake, with some providing only calories whilst others, in addition to calories, containing proteins, vitamins and minerals. Some can be added to the client's normal diet (for example powdered glucose polymers such as Polycal and Maxijul) and others are drinks that the client has between meals (for example Fresubin, Fortisip and Enlive). A dietician will prescribe the most appropriate supplements for the client following a nutritional assessment.

The client's cultural and religious beliefs also need to be considered when assisting the client to choose their meals. All hospitals are now required to provide special diets such as halal meals for Muslim clients as well as cater for vegetarians and vegans (see Table 5.2). However, it must be recognized that the choice available for these clients can be restricted.

Selection of appropriate fluids

As well as the client's food intake the health care professional needs to ensure that sufficient fluid is consumed on a daily basis. The normal requirement for an adult is three litres of fluid every 24 hours. Our role is to ensure that clients drink a sufficient amount of fluids to prevent dehydration. Encouraging patients to drink (or 'push fluids' as it is often known) is usually left to junior or inexperienced staff. It is therefore essential to have sound knowledge of the client's needs and to work very closely with them in order to encourage them to drink. They should be checked frequently, that is, at least every two hours, ensuring that they are offered the most acceptable beverages or alternatives (for example ice lollies) and that what the client has consumed is accurately documented.

An important point to remember is that some patients may have restrictions placed on the amount of fluid they are allowed to drink each day. For example, some clients with renal failure can be restricted to as little as 600 ml per day. Clients suffering from heart failure may also have restrictions on the amount of fluid they are able to receive. In contrast, clients may need extra fluid if they are losing excess fluid due to, for example, a raised temperature (pyrexia). It is therefore important to be aware of the client's individual hydration needs in order to educate and assist clients to select the appropriate amount and type of fluid.

In addition, the older person, children, people with learning difficulties and some clients with mental health problems can easily become dehydrated if they are not encouraged to drink sufficient amounts of water.

Monitoring nutritional status

To ensure that individual nutritional and hydration needs are sufficiently met some clients may need close and accurate monitoring. Nutritional assessment, as with other assessments, should not be a one-off process but continuous, especially those clients who are at risk of malnutrition. Simple indicators such as regular weighing and BMI calculations may be sufficient as long as the equipment used is accurate and of course available. It must be remembered, however, that short-term losses and gains will only reflect body fluid changes.

Another way of checking whether a client is eating a balanced diet is to get them to keep a food diary and then compare it to the ideal 'tilted plate' (see Figure 5.3). The more information that can be gained, the more

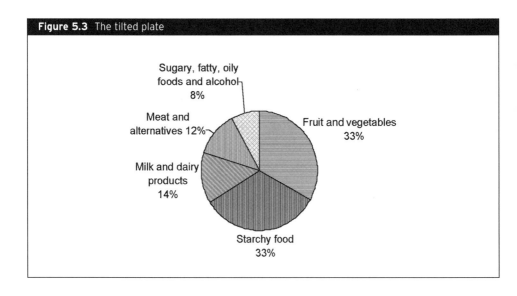

Figure 5.3 The tilted plate

Sugary, fatty, oily foods and alcohol 8%

Meat and alternatives 12%

Fruit and vegetables 33%

Milk and dairy products 14%

Starchy food 33%

accurate the resulting baseline will be. Food intake charts (see Figure 5.4) can be used. They are completed over several days to allow for any day-to-day fluctuations. Everything a client eats or drinks should be recorded, no matter how small the amount, for example three teaspoons of omelette. The important thing is that they are completed accurately and that they are evaluated by someone with sufficient knowledge to interpret the findings and ensure they are acted upon.

Figure 5.4 Food intake chart

Time	Food intake	Amount taken	Dietician's use	
			kcal	Protein
Breakfast	• Water	150 ml		
	• Tea, milk, 1 sugar, 2 scoops Polycal	175 ml		
	• White bread, butter & marmalade	1 slice		
	• Fruit juice	200 ml		
Mid-morning	• Tea, milk, 1 sugar, 3 scoops Polycal	150 ml		
Lunch	• Corn-beef hotpot	1 teaspoon		
	• Mash potatoes	2 teaspoons		
	• Bread & jam	½ slice		
	• Tea, milk, 1 sugar	150 ml		
	• Sponge & custard	4 teaspoons		
Mid-afternoon	• Tea, milk, 1 sugar, 3 scoops Polycal	175 ml 100 ml		
Evening meal	• Fortisip	100 ml		
	• Omelette	3 teaspoons		
	• Fortified soup	100 ml		
	• Water	100 ml		
Bedtime	• Fortisip	100 ml		
TOTAL				

The key features to check are the protein and calorie intakes, for example:

- Male clients aged 19–50 years should receive 2550 kilocalories and 55.5 g of protein daily.
- Female clients aged 19–50 years should receive 1940 kilocalories and 45 g of protein daily.

Monitoring fluid intake

As discussed, even minor changes in the body's fluid balance at cellular level can have serious consequences for the client's health. The health professional's role is critical in ensuring that fluid balance is monitored and recorded if the client is identified as:

- being at risk of dehydration
- having excessive fluid losses (e.g. diarrhoea)
- being fasted
- vomiting
- having fluid restriction
- being given any form of artificial nutrition or hydration
- or having some other condition which requires the fluid intake to be carefully maintained.

Therefore the total intake and output of fluids should be recorded on a fluid balance chart (see Figure 5.5).

Fluid balance charts

Each hospital or care facility will have its own form of fluid balance chart but they will all follow a similar format, requiring the nurse to record all types of fluid input and output, including:

- oral fluids
- enteral feed
- intravenous fluids
- blood and plasma
- urine
- vomit
- wound drainage
- nasogastric aspirate
- diarrhoea.

Figure 5.5 Fluid balance chart

Name: Date:

Time	Intake				Output			
	Intravenous fluid	Peg/parenteral nutrition	Oral intake		Vomit/gastric aspirate	Urine	Drains	Stoma
				cum. total				cum. total
01								
02								
03								
04								
05								
06								
07								
08								
09								
10								
11								
12								
13								
14								
15								
16								
17								
18								
19								
20								
21								
22								
23								
24								
TOTAL								

Total intake = ...Total output = ...

Instructions

Oral fluid...Dietary intake ....

You should always explain to the client why the recording is necessary and what the client is required to do (for example collecting and measuring urine) when you need to observe and record the nature and quantity of both input and output. The fluid balance chart should be assessed at regular intervals so that the input can be adjusted as required or abnormalities detected and reported promptly. Accurate recording of both intake and output is essential to be able to calculate the fluid balance correctly. The fluid balance should be totalled at the end of each 24-hour period and care needs reassessed.

Assisting with eating and drinking

In many acute hospitals domestic or housekeeping staff now serve meals but it is still essential that nurses supervise mealtimes to ensure that clients receive adequate amounts of the correct diet, that they eat it and that an evaluation is completed if any problems arise.

Unfortunately, food and drink is sometimes left out of reach, or the client is not given any help when required, resulting in the client receiving neither. Nutritional assessment should identify those people who need assistance with feeding. Guidance in assisting adults to meet their nutritional needs is given below. Assisting with feeding the client orally will be discussed in detail later in the chapter. Clients with special feeding needs such as enteral feeding via nasogastric or gastrostomy tubes have different needs and this is beyond the scope of this text.

In relation to infants the procedure for giving a bottle feed varies from hospital to hospital. Some have feed units where formula feeds are prepared and pasteurized centrally, thus preventing the need to make up feeds in ward kitchens. If you are required to prepare a formula feed, the manufacturer's instructions should be followed strictly, as the wrong concentration of powder to water can cause too-high sodium levels and be very dangerous to the infant. All the equipment to be used must be sterilized prior to undertaking the procedure, in keeping with local policy. Most acute hospitals have 'ready to feed' bottles of formula whereby a disposable teat is screwed onto the bottle and all that is required is to heat the feed to the correct temperature prior to giving. A full assessment is essential as some infants prefer the milk to be very warm and others just aired.

It is common for infants to have a small vomit when bringing up wind. This is known as a posit and is quite normal. There are various ways of helping the infant to bring up wind but placing the baby upright and rubbing or patting the back is a general recommended principle.

It is also recommended that weaning is introduced at 4 months of age and usually begins by introducing a few spoonfuls of baby rice mixed with breast milk or formula feed. Children should never be forced to eat, as this is often a cause of feeding problems such as food refusal later. It is normal for children to refuse food when they are ill or stressed. When feeding children the following foods should be avoided:

- under 3 years: nuts and nut products (can cause choking and are a potential allergen)
- under 1 year: nuts and nut products (as above); milk as a main drink (non-modified protein and therefore difficult to digest at this age); and added salt or sugar (can cause electrolyte imbalance)

- under 6 months: nuts and nut products (as above); milk as a main drink (as above); added salt or sugar (as above); fish, wheat, eggs (potential allergens), food with lumps in (potential for choking), and fresh fruit juices, which can cause diarrhoea if given in excess.

It should be remembered that mealtimes can also be used as teaching opportunities for children and other people with learning needs. In addition people with eating disorders may have individualized feeding programmes.

Eating and drinking also have a sociable element so it can sometimes be beneficial to involve relatives and friends in assisting clients to eat and enjoy their food, though this should be considered carefully beforehand, preferably in discussion with the client, as too many distractions can result in some clients being put off their food.

Clients, if able, may also benefit from being encouraged to eat in a separate dining area if one is available. This is especially pertinent in long-term care facilities and can also act as a useful reminder to those with limited memory who simply forget to eat without the external prompt of seeing others doing it. However, it may be more appropriate with clients who have difficulty feeding themselves, or those who need to be fed, to undertake this activity in more private surroundings in order to reduce embarrassment and distractions. What is important is that clients are involved in decisions about their food – its amount, timing and so on.

The aim of assisting clients with eating and drinking is to ensure that they receive the optimum amount of food and fluid whilst promoting independence. The following should be taken into account when preparing to assist clients:

- Consider the cleanliness of the surroundings and ensure that there are no unpleasant odours or sights.
- Remove any offensive material such as sputum pots, urinals, etc. from the client's bed table/eating area and clear a space for the tray.
- Place a chair beside the client's bed/chair for the nurse.
- Have to hand:
  non-slip plate mat
  plate guard
  appropriate handled cutlery or soft spoon in the case of children.
  (You may need to liaise with the occupational therapist to determine appropriateness of the above.)

The procedure for assisting is given below.

Procedure	Rationale
Wash hands following correct procedure, put on appropriate coloured apron, and ensure client has also washed their hands	To prevent cross-infection
Ensure that the client is in a comfortable position, preferably upright and sitting out of bed in a comfortable chair drawn up to a table of comfortable height	Sitting the client as upright as possible allows the first third of the oesophagus to work, generating a wave of peristalsis that takes food and fluid into the stomach and also lessens the risk of food passing into the respiratory tract
Tell the client what the choices of food are and ensure that an appropriate size meal is served	Gives client food choices. Some clients with a poor appetite can be overwhelmed if served a large portion
Before mealtimes avoid procedures that may result in the client being frightened, nauseated or in pain	To avoid stimulation of the GI tract by the sympathetic nervous system, as stimulation may decrease gut motility and also dry up secretions, resulting in a dry mouth and leaving clients unable to utilize what is taken in
Ensure that the food is presented attractively	To tempt the client's appetite
Make sure that the food is within reach of the client and that any packaged (e.g. butter, yoghurts, cartons, etc.) are opened if the client is unable to do so themselves	To ensure food is accessible to client
If the client is visually impaired make them aware of the position of the food on the plate, using the clock method to explain	To aid client to locate different foods, e.g. meat is at 12 o'clock, the vegetables are at quarter past and quarter to the hour, and the potatoes are at the half-past position
Provide a napkin	To protect the client's clothing
Provide the correct equipment, e.g. appropriate handled cutlery, plate guard, non-slip mat, for clients who are unable to grip normal cutlery, can only use one arm or have erratic hand and arm movement	To aid clients who are unable to grip normal cutlery. To prevent food from being pushed over the side of the plate. To prevent the plate from moving around
Cut up food as necessary	To promote independence
Encourage clients to eat and drink but do not press this if they indicate they have had sufficient	Small amounts taken more frequently may be more successful

Procedure	Rationale
After the meal, remove tray and crockery and wipe up any spillages	Infection control and to maintain a pleasant environment
Following eating, assist client to complete oral hygiene and wash hands/face as necessary	To meet client's hygiene needs
Put the client's belongings and a drink of water back within easy reach	To restore the client's environment
Wash hands and remove apron	Infection control
Complete documentation, e.g. food chart, fluid balance chart	Legal requirement to maintain documentation and safeguard client through good communications

Feeding dependent clients and clients with potential swallowing difficulties

Due to physical impairment, swallowing difficulties or generalized weakness some clients may be unable to feed themselves without assistance. In addition, some clients with severe dementia can also require assistance as they may not recognize food or cutlery or remember how to feed themselves. Having to be fed can threaten the client's dignity; therefore the health care professional should try to minimize any negative aspects that may contribute to these feelings. Therefore in addition to the guidelines outlined above, the procedure outlined below may also need to be considered.

The aim of feeding dependent clients is to ensure that they receive the optimum amount of food and fluid whilst maintaining their dignity and safety.

Procedure	Rationale
Wash hands following correct procedure and put on appropriate coloured apron, and also assist the client to wash their hands	Infection control
Ensure that the client is in a comfortable position, preferably upright and sitting out of bed in a comfortable chair drawn up to a table of comfortable height	Sitting the client as upright as possible allows the first third of the oesophagus to work, generating a wave of peristalsis that takes food and fluid into the stomach and also lessens the risk of food passing into the respiratory tract

Procedure	Rationale
If clients are unable to get out of bed ensure they are sat upright if condition allows; pillows should be arranged so that they can lean forward	As above
Put adjustable chairs into the upright position for meals and drinks and do not put back to recline position for at least 15 minutes afterwards	To prevent reflux of gastric contents
Ensure that the client can close their lips	A lip-seal needs to be maintained to trigger a swallow
Sit down at the same level to feed the client	Demonstrates a relaxed approach and that you can spend time with the client
Protect the client's clothing with a napkin	Maintains dignity
Ask the client in what order they would like the food	Client's likes/dislikes are met
Talk to the client but avoid asking questions during mealtimes	To avoid distracting the client during mealtimes
Allow time for the client to chew and swallow the food and drink before offering the next mouthful	To prevent client from feeling hurried as this could result in discouraging the client from eating
Adjust the amount of food and drink offered to suit client – a teaspoon per mouthful is plenty, and is best placed in the stronger side of the mouth	As above. Lessens risk of aspiration and choking
Allow two swallows per mouthful	Ensures mouth is empty
After every few mouthfuls ask the client to cough and to do so again at the end of the meal	To check and clear the airway
When giving a drink, tip the cup gently or use a feeder cup	Ensures flow of fluid is controlled and regulated. Lessens risk of aspiration and choking
With a napkin remove any dribbles of food or drink from the client's chin	To maintain client's dignity

Procedure	Rationale
During feeding listen to the client's voice by asking them to say 'Ah' after every few mouthfuls and if the client's voice sounds 'wet' or 'gurgly' **stop** feeding and call for qualified assistance	A wet or gurgly-sounding voice is a sign of aspiration into the respiratory tract
After the meal is completed check the mouth for retained food and remove it with a swab or toothbrush	To prevent aspiration and choking on retained food particles
Observe for any signs of choking, for example coughing or poor colour, and **stop** feeding immediately if this is suspected (refer to section below on choking)	To minimize harm

Further points

When feeding dependent clients and clients with potential swallowing problems consider the following:

- If a hot drink is delivered too early, put a lid on it and check it again later.
- A straw may be used to assist a client to drink. However, some clients may not be able to use a straw if their orbicularis oris muscle (the muscle around the mouth) is weak, as in some stroke patients, because it makes their suction power lower; straws with valves or a feeder cup may help.
- Some clients who cannot communicate their needs may go red in the face after meals, which may indicate that they need to defecate as a result of the gastrocolic reflex (putting food in at the top causes the system to shunt into action).
- All clients with problems swallowing must be referred to a speech and language therapist.
- The easiest consistency to eat is a smooth texture. Soft solids such as ice cream, yoghurt, custard and mashed potato are acceptable. Normal solids and thickened liquids are more difficult. These include thick milkshakes, yoghurt drinks and thickened soups.
- *Note*: It is important that the dietician in consultation with the speech and language therapist prescribes the appropriate diet after assessing the client, and you should therefore seek their guidance on the use of thickening powders etc. before you use them.

- Food types to be avoided by the client with eating or swallowing difficulties are those which are stringy, crumbly, tough, or of mixed textures (solids and fluids) or such things as chips, peas and sweetcorn.

Providing first aid to a client who is choking

In clients who are choking it is essential to remove the obstruction and clear the airway to prevent asphyxia.

Adult

If blockage of the airway is only partial, the client will usually be able to clear it by coughing so should be instructed to do so; but if obstruction is complete, urgent intervention is required to prevent asphyxia. Therefore if the client is conscious and breathing, despite evidence of obstruction:

Encourage them to continue coughing, but do nothing else.

If obstruction is complete, or the client shows signs of exhaustion or becomes cyanosed but *is still conscious, carry out back blows* as explained below.

Procedure	Rationale
Remove any obvious debris or loose teeth from the mouth	To clear airway of observable blockages and prevent inhalation of debris/teeth
Stand to the side and slightly behind client, support their chest with one hand and lean them well forward	To ensure that when obstructing object is dislodged it comes out of the mouth rather than going further down the airway
Give up to five sharp blows between the scapulae (shoulder blades) with the heel of your other hand; each blow should be aimed at relieving the obstruction, so all five need not necessarily be given	To dislodge the obstruction
If back blows fail, carry out abdominal thrusts: Stand behind the client and put your arms around the upper part of the abdomen	Correct position to administer abdominal thrusts

Procedure	Rationale
Make sure the client is bending well forwards	To ensure that when the obstructing object is dislodged it comes out of the mouth rather than goes further down the airway
Clench your fist and place it between the umbilicus (navel) and xiphisternum (bottom tip of the sternum) and grasp it with your other hand	To ensure correct hand position
Pull sharply inwards and upwards	To dislodge the obstructing object
If the obstruction is not relieved, recheck the mouth for any obstruction that can be reached with a finger, and continue alternating five back blows with five abdominal thrusts	To dislodge the obstructing object
If the client at any time becomes unconscious, carry out the following sequence of life support (see Chapter 1): Open the client's airway and remove any visible obstruction from the mouth.	To facilitate respirations
Check for breathing by looking, listening and feeling	To establish whether respiration has ceased. If not breathing, attempt to give two rescue breaths. Expelled air will enter client's lung fields, providing some oxygen
If effective breaths can be achieved within five attempts check for signs of a circulation and start chest compressions as given in Chapter 4 and/or rescue breaths as appropriate	See Chapter 4
If effective breaths cannot be achieved within five attempts: Start chest compressions immediately and do not check for signs of circulation.	To relieve obstruction and continue resuscitation
After 15 compressions **check the mouth for any obstruction** then attempt further rescue breaths.	Obstruction may have been dislodged by chest compressions
Continue to give cycles of 15 compressions followed by attempts at rescue breathing	To sustain circulation of blood during cardiac arrest - see Chapter 4

Procedure	Rationale
If at any time effective breaths **can** be achieved: • Check for signs of a circulation • Continue chest compressions and/or rescue breaths as appropriate	If obstruction is dislodged quickly a spontaneous circulation **may** return

Child and infant

If a child is breathing spontaneously, his/her own efforts to clear the obstruction should be encouraged. Intervention is necessary only if these attempts are clearly ineffective and breathing is inadequate.

- Do not perform blind finger sweeps of the mouth or upper airway as these may further impact a foreign body or cause soft tissue damage.
- Use measures intended to create a sharp increase in pressure within the chest cavity (an artificial cough), such as those procedures outlined below.

Procedure	Rationale
Perform up to five back blows: • Hold the child in a prone position and try to position the head lower than the shoulders with the airway • Deliver up to five smart blows to the middle of the back between the shoulder blades • If this fails to dislodge the foreign body proceed to chest thrusts	To dislodge the obstruction by creating a sharp increase in pressure within the chest cavity – an artificial cough

Perform up to five chest thrusts:
• Turn the child into a supine position, again with the head lower than the shoulders and the airway in an open position
• Give up to five chest thrusts to the sternum:
    The technique for chest thrusts is similar to that for chest compressions (see Chapter 4)
    Chest thrusts should be sharper and more vigorous than compressions and be carried out at a rate of about 20 per minute
	As above

Check mouth: • After five back blows and five chest thrusts check the mouth • Carefully remove any visible foreign bodies	Foreign object may have been dislodged

Procedure	Rationale
Open airway: • Reposition the airway by the head tilt and chin lift manoeuvre • Reassess breathing (refer to Chapter 1)	To facilitate respiration or to establish whether spontaneous respirations have ceased
If the child is breathing: • Turn the child into the recovery position • Check for continued breathing	To maintain airway and monitor respirations
If the child is not breathing: • Attempt up to five rescue breaths (refer to Chapter 1) to achieve two effective breaths, each of which make the chest rise and fall. The child may be apnoeic or the airway partially cleared; in either case the rescuer may be able to achieve effective ventilation at this stage • If the airway is still obstructed repeat the sequence as follows:	

For a child:
• Repeat the cycle previously outlined but substitute five abdominal thrusts for five chest thrusts:
   Use the upright position if the child is conscious; kneel behind a small child
   Unconscious children should be laid supine and the heel of one hand placed in the middle of the upper abdomen
• Alternate chest thrusts and abdominal thrusts in subsequent cycles
• Repeat the cycles until the airway is cleared or the infant breathes spontaneously
	To dislodge obstruction

For an infant: • Abdominal thrusts are not recommended in infants as they may rupture the abdominal viscera • Perform cycles of five back blows and five chest thrusts only	
Repeat the cycles until the airway is cleared or the infant breathes spontaneously	

Source: Resuscitation Council UK (2000) and reproduced with the kind permission of the Vice-Chairman.

If the infant or child stops breathing follow the BLS algorithm as outlined in Chapter 4.

It is important to stay with the client following any successful first aid measures, to provide reassurance and to address any further concerns or worries they may have; always ensure that the client is safe from further danger before leaving.

References and further reading

Allison S (1999) Hospital food as treatment. A report of a working party of the British Association of Enteral and Parenteral Nutrition. London: BAPEN.

Alzheimer's Society (2000) Food for Thought. London: Alzheimer's Society.

Anderson P (2000) Tickling patients' taste buds. Nursing Times 96(50): 24-6.

Association of Community Health Councils of England and Wales (1997) Hungry in Hospital. London: ACHEW.

Baillie L (2001) Developing Practical Nursing Skills. London: Arnold.

BAPEN (1996) cited in Freeman L (2002) Food record charts. Nursing Times 98(34): 53-4.

BAPEN (2000) Guidelines for the Detection and Management of Malnutrition in the Community. Maidenhead: BAPEN.

Barusi ME (1997) Human Nutrition: A Health Perspective. London: Edward Arnold.

Bond S (ed) (1997) Eating Matters. University of Newcastle: Health Service Research.

Brooker C (1998) Human Structure and Function, 2nd edn. London: Mosby.

Campbell J (1993) The mechanics of eating and drinking. Nursing Times 89(21): 32-3.

Cortis JD (1997) Nutrition and the hospitalised patient: implications for nurses. British Journal of Nursing 6(12): 666-74.

Davies S (1999) Dysphasia in acute strokes. Nursing Standard 13(30): 49-55.

Department of Health (2001) The Essence of Care. London: Department of Health.

Edwards S (1998) Malnutrition in hospital patients, where does it come from? British Journal of Nursing 7: 954-74.

Ferguson M, Capra S, Benner J, Banks M (1999) Development of a valid and reliable screening toll for adult hospital patient. Nutrition 15(6): 458-64.

Fieldhouse P (1995) Food and Nutrition Customs and Culture, 2nd edn. London: Chapman and Hall.

Hogston R, Simpson PM (1999) Foundations of Nursing Practice. Basingstoke: Macmillan.

McLaren S (1998) Nutritional screening and assessment. Professional Nurse (study supplement) 13(6): 59-65.

Micklewright A (1997) Good old home cooking. Nursing Times 93(49): 58-9.

Pender F (1994) Nutrition and Dietetics. Edinburgh: Campion Press.

Resuscitation Council UK (2000) Basic Life Support Resuscitation Guidelines 2000. http://www.resus.org.uk (accessed 5 January 2003).

Rollins H (1997) Nutrition and Wound Healing. Nursing Standard 11(51): 49-52.

Statutory Instrument No. 1455 (1989) Competencies for pre-registration nursing programmes. Approved Amendment No. 9, 18A. Nurses: Midwives and Health Visitors Rules.

Townely R, Robinson C (1997) Comfort eating. Nursing Times 93(94): 74.

Webb PG (2002) Nutrition: A Health Promotion Approach, 2nd edn. New York: Oxford University Press.

Chapter 6

Communicating

Penelope Ann Hilton and Helen Taylor

Introduction

Communication skills form the basic building bricks of all human interaction, be it a simple greeting or a complex relationship. Our verbal and non-verbal messages create pictures of who we are, how we are feeling and what we like or dislike. As health care professionals the pictures that we paint can reassure people and put them at their ease or, conversely, cause stress and anxiety and make them feel very vulnerable, uncomfortable or even, on occasions, aggressive. The development of sound therapeutic communication skills is therefore vital if we are to put people at their ease and make them feel secure, confident and valued. This means paying attention not only to what we say and do but also to how we say and do it.

Written communication skills are equally important. Clear and concise writing skills are essential not just for communicating effectively within a multidisciplinary team and ensuring consistent, quality care, but also to comply with the legal requirement to maintain comprehensive client care records.

Communication is, however, a two-way process. To communicate effectively means developing good skills at a personal level not only as a messenger, but also as a receiver. This requires us to listen attentively, be knowledgeable about the other person(s)'s abilities and perspectives as well as our own, and to develop the skills necessary to facilitate communication for those who are less able than ourselves, whatever the reason. For example, an individual with a specific learning difficulty may find it very difficult to verbalize their care needs and may need to use alternative modes of communication such as sign language to converse with us. A child may not yet have developed an understanding of the double entendres of some of our words. Clients who may be in pain or distress or those who are newly bereaved may find it exceptionally difficult to express their feelings and may ultimately need encouragement and support to do this.

Well-developed communication skills are therefore essential tools for nurses and other health care professionals, yet there is a plethora of literature that illustrates that we are notoriously poor at this activity for a variety of reasons, not least a perceived lack of time.

The factors that affect communicating may be:

- *physical* arising from alteration in the structure, function or process of the organs involved in communicating, such as damage to the tongue or larynx (voice box), or nerves supplying it
- *psychological* such as fear, anxiety and stress
- *sociocultural* including language, vocabulary, jargon and gesticulations
- *environmental*, for example poor lighting, noise or intrusions
- *politico-economic*, for instance type of occupation, neighbourhood

To help you to improve your communication skills and raise your level of awareness, this chapter offers guidance in relation to assessing an individual's ability to communicate, outlines some of the barriers to effective communication, and is followed by sections on how to respond appropriately to telephone calls, strategies to enable more effective communication with clients, and pointers for managing actual or potential violent or aggressive situations. A section on record keeping is also included.

The chapter is not intended to form a text on the theories of communication and consequently a comprehensive reading list, which includes some classic texts, is offered at the end of the chapter to help you direct your studies further. The reader is reminded that Chapter 7 offers more specific direction on how to communicate with clients who are dying and their significant others.

Common terminology

Active listening	Making a concerted effort to hear and understand the message the other person is trying to convey
Aggression	An attitude of hostility
Assertiveness	Able to assert or stand up for oneself
Attention	Awareness, mental concentration
Aural	Related to hearing
Clarifying	Making clear, ensuring understanding
Cognition	Ability to understand
Colloquialism	Word or phrase used in everyday speech but not for formal speech or writing
Communication	Passage of information from one to another
Cues	Things that are said or done which serve as a signal for something else to be done

De-escalation	A term commonly used to refer to techniques for diffusing a potentially aggressive or hostile situation
Double entendres	Double meanings dependent on context, for example 'The dog had to be put to sleep' and 'The anaesthetist will put you to sleep'
Dyslexia	Impairment of ability to read with comprehension
Dysphasia	Difficulty with speaking
Dysphonia	Difficulty in pronouncing sounds
Dyspraxia	Difficulty in performing co-ordinated movements
Empathy	The ability to identify with another person and understand their point of view
Inferences	To imply or suggest without stating directly
Labelling	A form of stereotyping, for example the unpopular patient
Mirroring	Unconsciously mimicking or adopting a similar position to another
Non-verbal communication	Communicating without the use of words, for example touch, gesture, facial expression
Oral	Related to mouth/speech
Paraphrasing	To express the meaning in simple terms, rewording
Perception	Ability to see and understand
Personality	Our individual character, our distinctive qualities which makes us who we are
Self-awareness	Noticing or being aware of yourself, your actions, your abilities and the impact these have or may have on others
Self-image	The way you see yourself or would describe yourself to others
Stereotyping	Assigning people to categories based on assumptions rather than fact, for example all fat people are lazy
Summarizing	Pulling together the main points
Sympathy	A feeling of pity or tenderness towards one who is suffering
Therapeutic	Healing, curative, comforting
Verbal communication	The spoken word and how we speak, including tone, pitch and volume
Validating	Confirming, checking
Violence	Unwarranted physical force or strength exerted with the intention of injuring or destroying another individual

Assessing the communication needs of clients

Remember that assessment of the activity of communicating is only part of a holistic nursing assessment and should not be undertaken in isolation without reference to or consideration of the client's other activities of living.

The specific points to consider when assessing a client's ability to communicate include:

- *Physical*
  Are their senses intact?
  Do they have any disorder or diseases affecting their sensory organs, for example laryngeal palsy, tinnitus, cerebral vascular accident (CVA)?
  Are they able to hear satisfactorily?
  Do they require any hearing aids? Are these functioning?
  How does the individual normally communicate: do they lip read, sign or Braille or use any speech aids such as a possum, robot or speaking tube?
  Do they have any speech impediment or impairment?
  Are they able to gesticulate, show affection or distaste?
  Can they control pitch and/or tone?
  Can they see satisfactorily or do they have/need spectacles or contact lenses?
  Can they read and/or write?
  Is their cognitive ability impaired?
  Are there any physiological signs of nervousness, for example dilated pupils, tremor, perspiration?

- *Psychological*
  Are they worried, nervous or frightened?
  Are they depressed, anxious or excitable?
  What is their level of intelligence?
  Can they understand complex language?
  What is their range of vocabulary?
  Are they self-confident/timid?
  Do they seem angry or upset? Are there any signs of actual or potential aggression or violence (see Chapter 6)?

- *Sociocultural*
  What is their first language or mother tongue?
  Do they possess a second or third language and if so how fluent are they?
  Do they understand the local dialect and colloquialisms?
  Are there any cultural issues surrounding communication and body language, for example social status, eye contact, proximity or touch?
  Do they use any unfamiliar jargon or abbreviations?
  Do they need an interpreter?

- *Environmental*
  Is the environment too hot, too cold or poorly ventilated?
  Is it too light or too dark?
  Does the client prefer a quiet environment or do they prefer background noise?
  Do they wish to communicate in a more private place or are they happy to discuss issues at the bedside in hearing distance of others?
  Are there any physical barriers to communication, for example furniture arrangement, size or type of room?
  Is the environment safe for client, self and others should the client become aggressive or violent?

- *Politico-economic*
  What communication channels does the individual use or prefer, for example telephone, newspapers, TV, email, Internet?
  Is the individual computer literate?
  Are they familiar with their rights/responsibilities, for example Data Protection Act?

Some of the barriers to effective communication are listed below:

- Failing to undertake a holistic assessment
- Failing to establish or explain the purpose of the interaction
- Failing to listen
- Failure to establish an environment of warmth and acceptance
- Personality, for example a person who is shy or introverted or, conversely, one who is domineering
- Lack of trust
- False reassurance
- Physical state, for example too tired or in too much pain
- Layout of furniture, for example sitting behind a desk or table
- Emotional state, for example too angry to listen
- Stress; seeming to be too busy
- Lack of privacy
- Visual impairment
- Environmental noise
- Hearing impairment
- Preoccupied
- Personal attitudes and values
- Status
- Religious/cultural beliefs
- Culture of the ward/institution
- Using closed questions inappropriately

- Using inappropriate language, colloquialisms and jargon
- Using leading questions inappropriately
- Misinterpreting or failing to clarify the essence of what has been or is being said
- Inappropriate use of facts
- Interrupting
- Not saying what you really mean
- Mode of dress, for example uniform, 'grunge'-look
- Standing over the person rather than being on the same level
- Missing verbal and non-verbal cues and inferences
- Giving advice
- Changing the subject
- Finishing sentences for clients
- Minimizing the other person's feelings
- Using trite expressions
- Jumping to conclusions
- Prolonged silence
- Probing.

Responding to telephone calls

Appropriate and effective responses to telephone calls promote good working relationships and engenders trust and confidence. The procedure that should be followed is given below.

Procedure	Rationale
In the clinical setting always try to answer the telephone within four rings	To reduce disturbance and prevent stress, as the most ill clients are normally placed nearest the nurses' station where telephones are situated
On answering greet the individual, give your location, designation and name, followed by an offer of assistance, for example 'Hello, Nightingale Ward, Staff Nurse Hilton, How can I help you?'	An initial greeting puts the person at their ease and can reduce tension. Giving your location reassures the caller that they have been connected to the correct location. When we communicate it is generally desirable to know with whom we are speaking. Offering assistance promotes confidence

Procedure	Rationale
Listen carefully to the message	To ensure understanding
Clarify the name of the caller, and, if appropriate, their designation if a member of staff, or their relationship to the client if it is an external enquiry	To protect client confidentiality
Remember to protect client confidentiality at all times. If you are unsure of the legitimacy of the caller ask for their telephone number and ring them back. If you are still unsure seek guidance from a more senior member of staff	To adhere to professional codes and local policy
If the caller is enquiring as to the health and welfare of a client, ensure that you obtain the client's consent before divulging any information	To prevent breach of client's rights
Communicate effectively, paraphrasing and clarifying as necessary	To ensure effectiveness
If you are unable to help the caller personally, offer to put them back to switchboard or put them in touch with another department or individual who may be able to help	To promote good relationships. A response of 'Oh they aren't here' or 'You've got the wrong department' is not particularly helpful and can increase tension and lead to unnecessary aggressive outbursts
If transferring the caller elsewhere give the caller the new number in case they are disconnected and advise them that this is a possibility	To reduce frustration and anxiety
If taking a message repeat the message back to the caller and ensure that the intended recipient receives the message promptly	To ensure effective communication
If a client enquiry, in settings where the handset is portable and the client well enough to receive calls, let the caller speak to the client personally	Increases feelings of worth and reduces the potential for misinterpretation
On completion of the call, document any necessary information clearly and promptly	To avoid miscommunication

Note that client confidentiality should be maintained at all times. Enquiries from the press or the police should *always* be referred to a senior member of staff or hospital administrator if in an institutional setting. Check your local policy.

Communicating with clients

It is important to remember that there is no substitute for face-to-face interaction, particularly on important issues, but only if this is undertaken with thought, using appropriate strategies following a full assessment of the client's ability to communicate.

Appropriate and effective communication helps to establish a therapeutic helping relationship, enables us to determine a client's care needs, promotes trust and confidence, and facilitates good multidisciplinary team working. Good practice is outlined below.

Procedure	Rationale
Prepare the environment, creating a climate of warmth and acceptance	To facilitate communication
Sit squarely in relation to the client, adopt an **O**pen posture, **L**ean in towards the client slightly, maintain comfortable **E**ye contact and **R**elax	The acronym SOLER, outlining 5 steps to good communication was first coined in the 1980s by Gerard Egan (2002) to help us to remember how using body position can improve our communication and help us to listen more effectively
Ensure that the client is comfortable, relaxed and if possible pain free and, if desirable and appropriate, arrange for a relative or significant other to be present	To promote client participation. To prevent misunderstandings and reduce the potential for collusion
If the content is likely to be of a confidential nature or has the potential to cause embarrassment find a private location acceptable to the client	To maintain confidentiality and self-esteem
Minimize the potential for interruptions	So that you can concentrate fully on the interaction
Review client information already available	To demonstrate good multidisciplinary team working
If possible, prepare what you want to say thoroughly beforehand	To keep the interaction focused
Determine how you are going to get your message across and how the client is going to communicate with you	Not all clients can hear or speak; it is therefore crucial that you establish effective means of communication. This may mean providing writing materials, arranging an interpreter or person to sign, or obtaining picture books, etc.

Procedure	Rationale
Make sure you allocate an adequate amount of time	To prevent you giving off a sense of urgency or rushing the client
Be prepared to adjust the time allowed if necessary	If the client is finding the interaction cathartic, they may open up about other issues. Whilst it may be appropriate to arrange a further meeting to discuss these or to refer the client to another party, sometimes the moment can be lost forever if the issue is not addressed at the time
Introduce yourself and address the client by their preferred name	Common courtesy
Explain the purpose of the interaction and encourage the client to partici-pate freely	Provides clarification and promotes equality
Check whether the client would like anyone else present	To provide support. **NB** If a non-consenting child, that is, one who is considered in law to be unable to legally give consent to care or treat-ment, it may be essential that a parent or guardian is present
Or conversely if anyone is present, does the client wish them to stay or leave?	To maintain privacy and confidentiality
Use questioning appropriately; ask one question at a time; give the client time to answer; use both open and closed questions; avoid questions such as 'Why?'	To avoid barriers to communication and to increase the likelihood that you elicit an appropriate response
Engage in active listening, displaying empathy and/or sympathy appropriately, and allow silence	To engender a sense of value, to demonstrate caring and to prevent misunderstanding
Keep your message simple – don't hide behind long words or jargon. Be clear, concise and completely honest	Helps gain the trust and confidence of the individual and ensure understanding
Use the full range of techniques such as:	To enhance the effectiveness of the interaction and ensure understanding
Clarifying observations and statements	If with a child, make sure you are aware of their understanding of different words to avoid anxiety and distress. For example, a child's understanding of 'being put to sleep' by the

Procedure	Rationale
Information giving Non-verbals, for example gestures, touch Paraphrasing Validating Summarizing	anaesthetist may be never waking up again, as recently happened to the pet dog. 'Stink coming' may mean they want to defecate. As you discover the child's range of vocabulary it is useful to document this in the care records to inform other members of the multidisciplinary team and prevent repetition
Be consistent	If you frequently change your mind or your views appear to conflict, this will weaken your message
Keep focused on current concerns	To avoid inappropriate distractions and therefore failings to achieve the purpose
If you promise to do something, make sure you deliver	Otherwise your credibility will be damaged
Provide opportunities for the client to ask questions	To decrease the potential for any feelings of powerlessness
Summarize the discussion and gain feedback from the client	To confirm understanding of the key points and to give a sense of closure
Record the interaction in the client's records and refer to a more senior member of staff or other agencies as appropriate	To promote multidisciplinary team working and continuity of care
If the communication has involved information giving, it is recommended that you also furnish the client with a copy of the information in written form following the interaction	To promote retention and sharing with significant others and to reduce potential misunderstanding and misconceptions

Managing violence and aggression

There are an increasing number of cases of aggressive incidents and physical assaults being reported in the media against health care personnel, suggesting that conflict and confrontation is occurring within a variety of clinical settings at a level previously unheard of. Whilst the potential for such conflict and confrontation can be minimized by developing effective interpersonal skills and adopting good communication strategies, it is perhaps inevitable, given the pain, stress and anxieties that many of our clients and their significant others have to face, that there will be occasions when tensions mount, leading to aggressive and/or violent outbursts.

Therefore, in order to remain safe, we need to remember 'the 4 A's':

Awareness	Be aware that the potential for conflict, confrontation or aggression may exist in the clinical area.
Alertness	Be alert to the potential for conflict within yourself, your clients and within the clinical environment itself.
Avoidance	Avoid a conflict situation if at all possible.
Appropriate response	If you cannot avoid the situation then have a considered and appropriate response to any signs of potential conflict or aggression.

Awareness and alertness

The ability to recognize that someone is getting angry involves us being able to pick up on the verbal and non-verbal clues that the other person is showing.

Some of the signs that might alert us to the fact that an individual is getting angry include:

- tapping fingers
- pacing around
- raised voice
- staring
- clenching fists
- swearing
- changing colour of face
- agitation
- finger wagging
- talking through clenched teeth.

Avoidance

There are many other signs that could alert us to the fact that someone is getting angry. Before we decide to get involved or deal with a situation, however, we need to assess the possible risks. In helping us determine whether or not we should avoid the situation Breakwell (1997) advises us to consider the following:

- Is the person I am dealing with facing high levels of stress?
- Is the person likely to be drunk or on drugs?
- Does the person have a history of violence?
- Does the person have a history of criminal convictions?

- Does the person have a history of psychiatric illness?
- Does the person suffer from a medical condition which may result in a loss of self-control?
- Has the person verbally abused me in the past?
- Has the person threatened me with violence in the past?
- Has the person attacked me in the past?
- Does the person perceive me as a threat to his/her children?
- Does the person think of me as a threat to his/her liberty?
- Does the person have unrealistic expectations of what I can do for him/her?
- Does the person perceive me as wilfully unhelpful?
- Have I felt anxious for my safety with this person before?
- Are other people present who will reward the person for violence?

These are seen as some possible predictors of the risk of violence in a situation and the more often you answer 'yes', the higher the risk.

Appropriate response

In any real-life situation we are rarely given the time to plan and carefully consider our actions prior to dealing with a conflict situation (unless we have deliberately provoked it!). Therefore, it is important that we consider this possibility beforehand and try to imagine how we might manage a conflict situation should it arise. This can help us identify the skills we have and what skills we need to develop, otherwise we may react to a situation in an entirely inappropriate way, which could actually make the situation worse.

Defusing an actual or potential situation

To calm an angry person we need to defuse the situation to make it less tense. A way to do this is to employ what are called de-escalation techniques. One model of de-escalation is called the 'Control Trilogy' (cited in Bibby, 1995). It has three stages: calming, reaching and controlling.

The calming stage

This involves keeping calm ourselves as well as endeavouring to calm the aggressor.

Calming self

Our ability to think can be affected by our emotional response to a situation, and in turn our emotional response can affect our behaviour. In a conflict situation emotions can run high; therefore it is important that we try to remain calm so that we can think clearly and act appropriately.

This is easier said than done when faced with an irate person, as it is a natural reaction either to want to move away and avoid the situation or to want to challenge the situation. In a clinical setting these options may not always be appropriate.

One technique we can use to calm ourselves is to breathe out slowly to a count of eleven and then to breathe in to a count of seven, repeating this for one or two minutes. Alternatively we can try tensing up our body muscles and then relaxing them. These techniques can be useful if you have the time to employ them. Remember that the angry person will also be picking up on your non-verbal behaviours.

Once confronted by the angry person, *listen* very carefully to what they have to say. The individual is most likely to be raising their voice in an effort to get their message across. It is our job to listen, both to the *content* and to the *emotion* of the message.

Listening carefully and not responding immediately also gives us time to compose ourselves as well as indicate to the other person that we are taking their complaint seriously. One possible reaction from the aggressor is to get more vocal or agitated or even violent if they believe that we are not listening to them or taking their complaint seriously.

There are several ways to demonstrate that you are interested and listening. Some verbal and non-verbal methods of communication that may assist you include:

- **Voice** - try to keep your voice calm and steady, talking slowly and clearly.
- **Face** - you can demonstrate that you are interested in the problem and willing to listen. Nod your head to show that you are listening.
- **Eyes** - establish eye contact to demonstrate your interest but avoid staring.
- **Position** - if possible establish yourself at the same level - try not to stand over them. Similarly it may be appropriate to stand up to demonstrate your attentiveness to their complaint.
- **Posture** - be aware of how you are presenting yourself. Avoid postures that might be interpreted as aggressive or defensive such as arms folded, pointing fingers or hands on hips.
- **Space** - angry people need more personal space so do not move too close to them - they may find this threatening or challenging.

Calming the aggressor

All of the above factors will help to present a calm demeanour and show interest in the angry person and their situation. This in itself may help to start to calm them down as they can tell that you are actively listening and no longer feel that they have to shout.

It can also have the effect of calming the person down by 'mirroring' or adopting a similar position to the other person. If our behaviour is calming and posing no threat or challenge then they also tend to relax a little and calm down.

Other things that you can do to calm the person down include:

- **Talking** – encourage them to keep talking. This may simply involve continuing as above to demonstrate that you are actively listening. Nod your head or prompt them verbally to expand further on the problem; this may involve asking them questions or asking them to explain.

- **Listening** – to their complaint/grievance as you will need to know all the facts or their perception of events. Listen to the emotions behind the complaint, what they are feeling. Note anything they say about their intentions.

- **Hearing them out** – do not try and hurry the conversation. Listen for as long as necessary, ensuring that they have the time and opportunity to say what they need to say. Do not try to draw conclusions yet.

- **Watching** – pay attention to both their verbal and non-verbal behaviour. Have their facial muscles relaxed? Is their body posture less confrontational? Are they breathing steadier? Has their voice lowered? These are some examples of evidence that they are calming down.

- **Resisting arguing** – do not try to challenge what the person is saying even if you know they are wrong. This will only serve to continue the conflict, or even escalate it, rather than defusing the situation.

- **Being yourself** – often angry people will verbally lash out at the nearest representative of the organization regardless of whether they have the responsibility for the problem or the authority to deal with it. Try and let them know who YOU are. Introduce yourself by name – try to convey yourself as an individual – not just 'one of them'. When things have calmed down sufficiently you can then explain your position and whether you or another member of staff are in a position to deal effectively with the problem.

- **Remaining calm** – don't be drawn into arguing back as this tends to make matters worse.

The reaching stage

This part of the de-escalation model is where, having encouraged the aggressor to air/explain their grievances, they are now calmer. This then gives us the opportunity to 'build bridges' and move the conversation forward.

Whilst continuing as before we need to:

- Clarify the facts or key points made, ensuring that you know exactly what the problem is or what is needed.

- Encourage further relaxation – perhaps by inviting them to sit down or offering refreshments – if it feels appropriate to do so.
- Demonstrate that you empathize with their feelings but avoid any verbal or non-verbal behaviour which they may consider to be patronizing.
- Keep encouraging the person to relate to you. If it feels safe and comfortable then move closer and perhaps alongside the person.
- Avoid jargon and use straightforward language, encouraging the individual to ask questions or to clarify any issues they have.

The controlling stage

Now that the person is calm and communicating normally, the final stage involves both parties working together to resolve the problem. If it is within your ability/responsibility/authority then continue as before and do the following:

- **Set targets** – together agree what needs to be done, by whom and when.
- **One at a time** – if the issue is not simple or there is more than one issue start with the simplest – any resolution will leave both feeling as though something has been achieved.
- **Be realistic** – both parties need to be clear and honest about what is realistically achievable and over what timeframe.
- **Admit mistakes** – if a mistake has been made then admit it but if the mistake is on the part of the angry person do not blame them or belittle them – it may be a simple case of misunderstanding.
- **Take your time** – ensure that the person does not feel rushed.
- **Do not use jargon** – this may confuse the person, make them feel more anxious or make them feel that you are patronizing them.
- **Get assistance** – if you are not able to solve the situation or are not in a position to be able to make decisions, seek assistance from a more senior member of staff. Do not make promises that you are unable to keep.
- **Recognize** – that not all problems can be solved immediately. You may need to get more facts or information before a decision can be made. Ensure that this is understood and then explain how you will then proceed and how you will give feedback to the person, and in what timeframe. Once you have given a commitment it is vital that you keep it.
- **Review** – reconsider the event. What resolution have you reached between you, who has agreed to do what, and when are you going to get back in touch and how? Report the incident and ensure that it is well documented. It may also be necessary to complete an incident form to inform your local risk-management strategy. Check your local policy.
- **Finally** – it is important to remember that, in these circumstances, it is the behaviour of the individual that is being rejected – not the person –

and they need to know this, as it is likely that you will need to continue to be involved in their care or that of their significant other.

Threat of physical attack

If at any time you feel physically threatened then listen to your instinct and get out of the situation immediately. You are not expected to deal with any physical altercation or to put your physical well-being at risk. If there is damage to or theft from the environment this can easily be repaired or replaced – you cannot.

Using physical force or restraint

The use of physical force or restraint is an action of last resort and in some cases it can be both dangerous and illegal. It is therefore essential that you consult with and adhere to local policies and procedures.

Record keeping

Written communication is as important in the health care arena as both verbal and non-verbal communication. Maintaining clear, concise but comprehensive client care records is absolutely essential both in terms of providing continuity of client care of a high standard and in terms of meeting legislative requirements.

Remember, in a court of law it is assumed that *if the care was not documented then it didn't happen.*

With the advent of information technology, computerized information systems are being increasingly used to record, store and evaluate information pertaining to clients. These are proving very useful in terms of easier and speedier access to information both within and across care environments, for example department to department, hospital and community. Whatever method is used in your area, however, it is important that you familiarize yourself with the systems and ensure that you do not breach client confidentiality.

The Nursing and Midwifery Council has adopted the standards for record keeping produced by their predecessors, the UKCC (1999). The main tenets are summarized below.

Client records should:

- be factual, consistent and accurate

- be written as soon after the event as possible and, if possible, with the involvement of the client
- be clear, legible and readable following photocopying
- be written in a manner that cannot be erased
- be timed, dated and signed with name printed by the side and indicating your role, for example *PA Hilton* (PA Hilton, Staff Nurse)
- be devoid of abbreviations, jargon or meaningless phrases such as 'Bed bath given'
- not contain any subjective, offensive statements or irrelevant speculation
- be written in a language understandable by the client
- identify client problems and steps taken to rectify them
- provide evidence of the care that has been planned and delivered
- include information that has been shared with others
- include evidence of evaluation of the efficacy of care delivery.

The frequency of entries is generally determined by local policies though this should be complemented by sound professional judgement. These standards do not just apply to care plans but are equally valid when recording observations and assessments on the multiplicity of charts that abound today.

The Access to Health Records Act (1990) and the Data Protection Act (1984) gives clients access to their health care records, whether held manually or on computer. The latter Act also regulates the storage and protection of client information held on computer. It is therefore worthwhile familiarizing yourself with these documents so that you are fully aware of clients' rights.

Finally, should you wish to access clients' records for research purposes, written approval must be obtained from your local research ethics committee. The use of client records to supplement summative assignments or other course work is considered a direct breach of client confidentiality and should therefore be avoided.

References and further reading

Argyle M (1989) Psychology of Interpersonal Behaviour, 2nd edn. Harmondsworth: Penguin.
Argyle M (1990) Bodily Communication, 2nd edn. London: Routledge.
Arnold E, Boggs KU (1999) Interpersonal Relationships: Professional Communication Skills for Nurses. London: Saunders.
Ashmore R (1999) Heron's intervention framework: an introduction and critique. Mental Health Nursing 19(1): 24-7.
Audit Commission (1993) What Seems to be the Matter. Communication between Hospitals and Patients. London: HMSO.

Berne E (1964) Games People Play. Harmondsworth: Penguin.

Bibby P (1995) Personal Safety for Health Care Workers. Aldershot: Ashgate.

Bradley JC, Edinberg MA (1990) Communication in the Nursing Context, 3rd edn. Norwalk: Appleton & Lange.

Breakwell GM (1997) Coping with Aggressive Behaviour. Leicester: BPS Books.

Burnard P (1997) Effective Communication Skills for Health Professionals, 2nd edn. Cheltenham: Stanley Thornes.

Burton R (1998) Violence and aggression in the workplace. Mental Health Care 2(3): 105-108.

Caris-Verhallen WMCM, Kerkstra A, Bensing JM (1997) The role of communication in nursing care for elderly people: a review of the literature. Journal of Advanced Nursing 25(5): 915-33.

Caris-Verhallen WMCM, Kerkstra A, BensingJM (1999) Non-verbal behaviour in nurse-patient communication. Journal of Advanced Nursing 29(4): 808-18.

Chant S, Jenkinson T, Randle J, et al. (2002) Communication skills: some problems in nursing education and practice. Journal of Clinical Nursing 11(1): 12-21.

Cooley D (2000) Communication skills in palliative care. Professional Nurse 15(9): 603-605.

Department of Health (1998) The New NHS Charter: A Different Approach. Leeds: NHS Executive.

Dreger V (2001) Communication: an important assessment and teaching tool. Insight 26(2): 57-62.

Duxbury J (2000) Difficult Patients. Oxford: Butterworth Heinemann.

Egan G (2002) The Skilled Helper, 7th edn. Pacific Grove, CA: Brooks & Cole.

Ellis RB, Gates RJ, Kenworthy N (1995) Interpersonal Communications in Nursing: Theory and Practice. Edinburgh: Churchill Livingstone.

Faulkner A (1998) Effective Interaction with Patients, 2nd edn. London: Churchill Livingstone.

French P (1994) Social Skills for Nursing Practice, 2nd edn. London: Chapman & Hall.

Garnham P (2001) Understanding and dealing with anger, aggression and violence. Nursing Standard 16(6): 37-42.

Hargie ODW (1997) The Handbook of Communication Skills. London: Routledge Press.

Heinekin J (1998) Patient silence is not necessarily client satisfaction: communication problems in home care nursing. Home Healthcare Nurse 16(2): 115-21.

Heron J (1990) Helping the Client: A Creative Practical Guide. London: Sage.

Hines J (2000) Communication problems of hearing impaired patients. Nursing Standard 14(19): 33-7.

Kagan C, Evans J (1995) Professional Interpersonal Skills for Nurses. London: Chapman & Hall.

Knapp M (1971) Non-verbal Communication in Human Interaction. London: Holt, Rhinehart & Winston.

Macmillan Open Learning (1997) Breaking down the barriers to effective communication. Nursing Times 93(2): 37-8.

Marland G (2000) Cognitive deficits in schizophrenia. Nursing Times 96(16): 43-4.

Mason T, Chandley M (1999) Managing Violence and Aggression. Edinburgh: Churchill Livingstone.

Mehrabian A (1969) Tactics in Social Influence. London: Prentice Hall.

Metcalfe D (1998) Doctors and patients should be fellow travellers. British Medical Journal 316(20): 1893.

Miller R (1990) Managing difficult patients. London: Faber & Faber.

Minard HA (1997) Communication in Health Care: A Skills Based Approach. Oxford: Butterworth.

Morcombe J (1999) Interpersonal approaches to managing violence and aggression. Emergency Nurse 7(1): 12-16.

Morrison P, Burnard P (1997) Caring and Communicating the Interpersonal Relationship in Nursing, 2nd edn. Basingstoke: Macmillan.

Nabb D (2000) Visitors' violence: the serious effects of aggression on nurses and others. Nursing Standard 14(23): 36-8.

Newell R (1994) Interviewing skills for Nurses and other Health Care Professionals. London: Routledge.

Nurses and Midwives Council (2002) Code of Professional Conduct. London: Nurses and Midwives Council.

Paterson B, Leadbetter D, McCornish A (1997a) De-escalation in the management of aggression and violence. Nursing Times 93(36): 58-61.

Paterson B, Tringham C, McCornish A, et al. (1997b) Managing aggression and violence: a legal perspective on the use of force. Psychiatric Care 4(3): 128-31.

Peplau H (1952) Interpersonal Relationships in Nursing. New York: GP Putnam.

Rader J (1994) To bathe or not to bathe: that is the question. Journal of Psychosocial Nursing 32(9): 53-4.

Reynolds W, Scott P (2000) Do nurses and other professional helpers normally display much empathy? Journal of Advanced Nursing 31(1): 226-34.

Rippon T (2000) Aggression and violence in health care professions. Journal of Advanced Nursing 31(2): 452-60.

Stirling C (2001) Physical Intervention in the management of aggression and violence: legal, professional and ethical considerations. Journal of Adult Protection 3(3): 30-40.

Stirling C, McHugh A (1998) Developing a non-aversive intervention strategy in the management of aggression and violence for people with learning difficulties using natural therapeutic holding. Journal of Advanced Nursing 27(3): 503-509.

Stockwell F (1984) The Unpopular Patient. London: Croom Helm.

Thomas B, Hardy S (1997) (eds) Stuart and Sundeen's Mental Health Nursing - Principles and Practice. London: CV Mosby.

Tingle JH (1998) Nurses must improve their record keeping skills. British Journal of Nursing 7(5): 245.

Tschudin V (1995) Counselling Skills for Nurses, 4th edn. London: Baillière Tindall.

Turnbull J, Patterson B (1999) Aggression and Violence: Approaches to Effective Management. London: Macmillan.

Tyrell M (2000) The prevention of aggression and violence in the accident and emergency department. Nursing Review 18(1): 14-18.

UKCC (1999) Standards for Record Keeping. London: UKCC.

Vanderslott J (1994) A positive exercise in damage limitation: management of aggression in elderly confused people. Professional Nurse 10(3): 150-2.

Villarruel AM, Portillo CJ, Kane P (1999) Communicating with limited English proficiency persons: implications for nursing practice. Nursing Outlook 47(6): 262-70.

Walker J (2002) Safety first. Nursing Times 98(9): 20-21.

Whittington R, Patterson P (1996) Verbal and non-verbal behaviour immediately prior to aggression by mentally disordered people: enhancing the assessment risk. Journal of Psychiatric and Mental Health Nursing 3(1): 47-54.

Whittington R, Wykes T (1996) An evaluation of staff training in psychological techniques for the management of patient aggression. Journal of Clinical Nursing 5(4): 257-61.

Williams D (1996) Communication Skills in Practice: A Practical Guide for Health Professionals. London: Jessica Kingsley.

Wondrak R (1998) Interpersonal Skills for Nurses and Health Care Professionals. Oxford: Blackwell Science.

Wykes T (1994) Violence and Health Care Professionals. London: Chapman and Hall.

Chapter 7

Dying

Penelope Ann Hilton

Introduction

From the moment we are born the only predictable event in life is that one day we will die. Dying is thus an inevitable part of life, yet it remains surrounded in mystery to a large extent, provoking fear and anxiety in most individuals, particularly in Western society. However, when explored, it is not usually the thought of death that creates anxiety but the where, the when, the why and the how. Other issues of concern often include: what will happen to my body; how will those left behind manage, financially and emotionally; and who will help them through this difficult time? It is also not unusual for dying clients to feel guilty about the distress they perceive they are causing to their loved ones.

Addressing such issues with clients and their relatives can be daunting for even the most seasoned health care professional, let alone the novice. Consequently, whilst this chapter aims to offer guidance for those with little or no experience of death and dying, the reader is reminded that it is important for us all to recognize and acknowledge our limitations and not be afraid to seek assistance if we are unsure or worried about any particular aspects of care delivery.

Factors affecting dying may be:

- *physical* arising from the nature of the terminal illness or cause of death such as pain, nausea, breathlessness
- *psychological* such as fear and anxiety about death itself or the effects on those left to grieve
- *sociocultural* including personal beliefs about death and attitude towards death and dying
- *environmental*, for example preferred place of death, quiet/noisy, private/open
- *politico-economic* such as lack of finances for funeral, outstanding debts.

This chapter outlines some of the principles and practices surrounding care of the dying and the performance of last offices. The need for respect of clients' and relatives' beliefs, values, culture and customs when initiating and carrying out these final acts of nursing care is emphasized throughout. The chapter includes sections on common terminology; communicating with dying clients; the signs of approaching death; informing relatives; confirmation of death; the equipment required to perform last offices; and the procedure for cleansing, dressing and positioning of the deceased, paying due regard to issues surrounding infection control, labelling of the body and care of the deceased's property and valuables. The reader is reminded of the need to refer to local policy and procedures throughout but particularly in relation to infection management and removal of the body from the clinical area. The chapter concludes with references and direction to enable further reading.

Common terminology

Cadaver	Corpse, dead body
Cheyne-Stokes respirations	Periodic breathing characterized by a gradual increase in respiration followed by a decrease in respiration resulting in apnoea
Coroner	A person appointed by the Home Office who is required by law to investigate deaths due to unnatural, suspicious or unknown causes
Inquest	An investigation held by the Coroner when death is known or suspected to be due to any other cause than natural death
Medical Certificate of Death	Sometimes referred to as the Death Certificate, it is a legal document required by the Registrar of Births, Deaths and Marriages before they can issue a form permitting disposal of the body
Palliative	Something which relieves discomfort or distress but does not cure
Pathologist	A doctor trained in the detection and diagnosis of disease
Post-mortem	Involves the examination of the brain and other internal organs by a pathologist, usually undertaken when the cause of death is uncertain or suspicious
Prognosis	Course of the disease including expected outcome
Rigor mortis	The term given to the stiffening of the body following death
Rose Cottage	A term commonly used for the mortuary when speaking in a public area

Assessing the dying client

Remember that assessment of the activity of dying is only part of a holistic nursing assessment and should not be undertaken in isolation without reference to or consideration of the client's other activities of living.

The specific points to consider when assessing the dying client are:

- *Physical*
  Is the client in any physical distress, for example nauseous, vomiting, dehydrated, breathless, constipated, unable to sleep, immobile, in pain?
  Is everything possible being done to promote the client's comfort?
  Could anything else be done?
  Do they have a 'Do not resuscitate' order and has this been discussed with the client and their next of kin?
  Can any other members of the multidisciplinary team offer help or guidance?
  Could any alternative therapies be of help?
  Are there any physical effects on family/friends?
  Is the client an actual or potential organ donor and are the family aware?
  Do the client/family wish sustained treatment?
  Remember, good symptom control is not just for clients but also for relatives, as they have to live with their memories.

- *Psychological*
  Are the client/family aware of the diagnosis/prognosis?
  What are the client/family's beliefs about death and dying?
  Are the client/relatives frightened, anxious, depressed?
  Do they have any concerns that can be addressed by you or others, for example a Macmillan nurse, the palliative care team?
  Is everything possible being done to promote the client's autonomy, privacy and dignity?
  Have they any outstanding or unfinished business they wish to address?
  Do they require you to contact any outside agencies on their behalf?
  What effect will the death have on family members?

- *Sociocultural*
  Do you have full contact details of next of kin/religious leaders?
  Do they wish to see a minister, priest or other religious leader?
  Do the client/family wish anyone else to be contacted?
  Do the client/family feel isolated?
  Does the client wish restricted or unrestricted visiting?
  Are family and significant others aware of the visiting agreement?
  Are there any other specific spiritual, religious or cultural wishes to be addressed before, during or following death? (see Table 7.1, p. 187)
  Do the client's family wish to be participants or observers of care?

If they wish to participate how can this be facilitated?

Are there any barriers preventing their involvement that can be over-come, for example lack of skill or knowledge?

Do relatives wish to be informed immediately if their loved one dies and they are not present? This is particularly important if the death occurs during the night, if the relatives live a long distance away, or the next of kin is ill or disabled.

Who should be informed of the death first?

- *Environmental*

  Does the client wish to die in a clinical environment, hospice or at home? Can this be facilitated?

  What support mechanisms are required/available?

  Is the environment of care conducive to the client/visitors? Could it be improved?

  Are there any concerns about necessary environmental changes that might be incurred for spouse/family following death?

- *Politico-economic*

  Have the client/relatives any financial worries or concerns?

  Could referral to other agencies help?

  Are there any other health or support services available for the dying or bereaved?

  Have they made a will? If not, how can this be facilitated, if desired?

Communicating with dying clients and their relatives

Dying clients and their relatives often have preconceived ideas and some-times misconceptions about death and dying. Whilst some individuals seek answers and reassurance from religious sources regarding the where, when, why and how death might befall them, many clients and their loved ones look to health care professionals. Unfortunately we are not always able to give an unequivocal response and often fear that anything we do say will create even greater anxiety and distress. Often we feel too uncomfortable with the topic ourselves to believe we can be of any help to others. Rather than admit these facts, all too frequently we adopt the tactic of self-preservation whereby we use a variety of strategies, consciously and sometimes unconsciously, in the hope of avoiding these difficult questions. The commonest strategy in busy health care environments is to focus on clients' physical needs and appear 'too busy to chat'. The consequence of such actions is that clients and their families are frequently left with unmet needs. The following section is therefore designed to offer some pointers for novice health care professionals when communicating with dying clients and their significant others.

Always remember, dying clients are, in fact, still very much alive and may not necessarily wish to be surrounded by those they perceive to be doom and gloom 'experts', nor wish any encounter to be planned like a military operation. They very often welcome the approach of bright-eyed, effervescent, naive neophytes so never be afraid to stop and talk to a client who is known to be dying: it can make such a difference to their last days, hours or moments of life. The greatest skill is recognizing when *they* wish to be left alone.

Before the interaction:

- Be clear about your own attitudes, values and beliefs about death and dying.
- Learn about and endeavour to be accepting of others' differing values and beliefs.
- Do not underestimate the importance of spirituality to some clients.
- Do not assume that because it is OK for you and your nearest and dearest that it will be OK for others.
- Be aware of the support mechanisms you can draw upon if you feel you are getting 'out of your depth', such as the Macmillan nurse, palliative care team, chaplaincy and specialist counselling services.
- Establish what has or has not been said by the doctors and other health care professionals.
- Establish whom the client wishes to be present during the interaction, taking care not to be drawn into any collusion or secrecy.
- For some clients tape-recording the interaction can be helpful to refer back to. They may then also share it with others if they so wish.
- If possible prepare the environment to ensure privacy and no disturbances (see Chapter 6).

At the commencement of the interaction:

- Try not to have any preconceived ideas: each client and relative is a unique individual and may respond very differently to similar sets of circumstances.
- Think before you open your mouth to speak.
- Establish the most important source of information to the client/family.
- Establish the client and family's level of awareness of the situation.
- Establish trust and confidence.
- Try not to be judgemental.
- Do not be afraid to stop and listen.

- Be accessible; show that you have time and are willing to listen.
- Don't be afraid to say 'I don't know'.
- Don't agree to collude or keep secrets.
- Be prepared for the vast array of reactions that can occur, such as anger, guilt, fear, denial, acceptance or loss of control.
- Sometimes anger can be directed at you; try not to appear defensive unless truly warranted. Don't take it personally. Try and stay calm and kind. Try to understand and to see the situation from their perspective. See Chapter 6 for guidance as to what to do should the situation become particularly aggressive or violent.
- Empathy in this situation is almost impossible, but sympathy and compassion can be equally important.
- Give time to grieve, talk, and reminisce, to express fears and anxieties, to express wishes and dreams.
- Offer to contact a priest or other religious leader if the client wishes.

At the end of the interaction:

- Ensure that the client and/or their relatives are clear about the key points of the interaction.
- If appropriate write down the key points for them to keep, refer back to and/or, if desired, share with others.
- If necessary arrange a day/time for a follow-up consultation.
- Make it clear that either you or a colleague are available at any time should the client require any further help or support.

Following the interaction:

- Document any key points that will facilitate continuity of care.
- If you have indicated that you will contact another person, health professional or agency, be sure to do so promptly before you become involved with other tasks that mean you might forget later.
- Endeavour to promote a positive atmosphere.
- Always convey the impression that you have time, and pay attention to the little things, as they often mean the most to clients and those they love (see Chapter 10).

Communicating with dying patients and their significant others is probably one of the hardest tasks facing health care professionals, but it can be one of the most rewarding. Do not be disheartened if you are left thinking you didn't get it quite right. It takes time to develop the skills. Instead analyse the interaction and discuss your thoughts and feelings with your mentor or other members of the health care team.

Signs of approaching death

It is not uncommon for novice health care professionals to be anxious about their first encounters with death. The following points may help to allay some of the anxieties you might have arising from a limited knowledge base, and reduce some of the fear stemming from the 'unknown'.

- As the client's bodily systems begin to shut down, motion and sensation are gradually lost.
- Whilst the client's temperature may be elevated they often feel cold and clammy to touch. This can be disconcerting for both relatives and staff and can be eased by regular cleansing with moist wipes.
- Respirations may be noisy due to the build-up of secretions in the lungs. This can be distressing for relatives and inexperienced staff. Administering an antimuscarine such as hyoscine butylbromide sublingually or intramuscularly, if prescribed, can sometimes reduce this.
- Cheyne-Stokes respirations are common and again can be disconcerting if not expected or understood.
- Circulation fails and the blood pressure falls. It is therefore best to remove any monitoring devices, which tend to alarm when pulse, blood pressure and/or respirations fall outside the parameters set.
- Pain, if it has been present, may subside. Unfortunately this can sometimes lure relatives into a false sense of security.
- The client's mental condition usually deteriorates though it is thought by many that hearing remains acute and indeed may be accentuated immediately prior to death.

Informing relatives

If relatives are not present the identified next of kin should be informed of the client's deteriorating condition. Only in exceptional circumstances should relatives be informed of a death over the telephone. An alternative solution, particularly for those next of kin who are immobile or live a considerable distance away, is to inform their local police force, who will usually deliver a 'death warning' in person and can thus assess the situation and provide support if necessary.

It is the responsibility of the senior nurse to contact relatives and ask them if they wish to attend. If you are asked to deputize and feel confident, knowledgeable and competent to do so you should:

- give name, title and where you are calling from
- determine the identity of the person to whom you are speaking
- explain that the client's condition has worsened

- stay calm and speak in a controlled manner
- use short sentences offering small pieces of information
- pause to allow the receiver of the call time to comprehend
- urge the individual to come to the hospital and reassure that care is being given. Ask if they require you to contact any other persons on their behalf such as a priest or other religious leader
- document time and nature of information given and the name of the recipient(s).

Helping arriving relatives

To avoid confusion, ideally the nurse who made the call should meet the relatives on arrival to provide continuity of care. They should not be left alone but shown to a private place.

Grief reactions may differ:

- be prepared and avoid being judgemental
- words of comfort are often difficult to find; sincerity is generally the best course of action
- active listening is often the best approach as this allows for reminiscing and/or expression of emotions.

Those receiving notification of a sudden unexpected death may show severe emotional reactions. Encouraging survivors to view the deceased can seem quite brutal; however, this can help to reinforce the reality of the event and assist subsequent grieving.

Consider the likely effect of showing personal emotion. It may or may not be appropriate depending upon the circumstances surrounding the actual/impending death.

Confirming death

Clients are usually pronounced dead by a doctor; however, some senior nurses may undertake this task as part of their expanded role if the death was expected and there are no suspicious circumstances. The procedure is usually performed when relatives are present though on occasions circumstances may prevent this.

Nurses and others may recognize classic signs, which are:

- no evidence of pulse, respirations or blood pressure
- pupils fixed and dilated.

Post-mortems may only be carried out with written consent of relatives *unless* the death occurs in suspicious circumstances or occurred without prior medical intervention. In these cases permission – whilst desirable – is not required in law. A booklet produced by the Royal College of Pathologists (2000), *Examination of the Body after Death*, offers useful information about post-mortem examination for relatives, and copies are readily available from http://www.rcpath.org.uk.

If a post-mortem is to be carried out, *under no circumstances* should any tubes, catheters or other invasive equipment be removed from the body. If unsure then you must check with the medical officer or senior nurse before performing Last Offices and adhere strictly to their guidance.

Accounting for valuables

- Be aware of local policy.
- All valuables should be identified, accounted for and sent for safe-keeping as soon as is reasonably practical, in keeping with local policy.
- Any jewellery left on the deceased should be taped, and details noted on the appropriate documentation.
- A second responsible person should always be called on as witness when accounting for client property whether the client is deceased or otherwise.
- No valuables or other client property should be given to relatives prior to full documentation and a signature of receipt should be obtained.
- It is usual to ask relatives to collect the deceased's belongings when they come to collect the Medical Certificate of Death. This allows time to parcel the property more appropriately and thus reduce the potential for further distress.

Last Offices

Specific needs in relation to Last Offices can vary according to the client's cultural and religious practices (see Table 7.1). It is therefore important to elicit the wishes of the client and of the relatives prior to death if at all possible, and to make sure that these wishes are clearly documented in the client's records and adhered to. Two staff working quietly together should normally undertake this procedure, paying due regard to legal require-ments including health and safety issues as appropriate (see 'Special precautions'). As a point of note, rigor mortis generally begins 2–3 hours following death; it is therefore advisable to perform Last Offices prior to this occurring, as movement and positioning will otherwise be impossible.

Some relatives may explicitly express a wish to undertake the Last Offices themselves, whilst others may wish to participate but are not aware of the possibility. Every effort should be made to elicit relatives' wishes in a tactful manner without creating a feeling of pressure. When relatives express such a desire this should, if at all possible, be facilitated, with both parties having a clear understanding of the desired degree of involvement. It is essential that client advocacy continues in death and every effort should be made to ensure continued privacy and dignity.

Table 7.1 Last Offices: special considerations for different cultural and religious practices

Religion	Special considerations
All denominations	Whilst the needs of all clients must be considered, visitors are generally extremely important to the dying and bereaved. Staff should therefore be sensitive to the needs of dying clients and their visitors, who may wish to chant, sing or pray, and facilitate this as much as possible but paying due regard to the needs of other clients.
Bahai	Relatives usually say prayers over the deceased prior to the performance of Last Offices, but it is generally acceptable for nursing staff to carry out the procedure itself. There are usually no objections to the carrying out of a post-mortem or to organ donation.
Buddhism	The body should not be moved for one hour following death. Some clients or relatives may request the presence of a Buddhist nun or monk. There are usually no objections to the carrying out of a post-mortem or to organ donation though some Far Eastern followers may object.
Christianity	Differing denominations follow differing customs but Last Offices as outlined in the text are generally acceptable. The client or relatives may wish the hospital chaplain or priest to perform the last rites, preferably prior to death. Sometimes relatives may wish to place a rosary, icon or flowers with the deceased and/or place the hands in prayer. Staff should not do this as a matter of course as some relatives find it very distressing, whilst others may consider it their personal right, responsibility or duty. Relatives may wish to undertake or participate in Last Offices. Post-mortem and organ donation are generally acceptable though some people may object depending on their individual socialization processes.
Christian Science	Last Offices as outlined here are acceptable, though female staff should handle a female body. Post-mortem and organ donation are acceptable if essential.
Hinduism	Distress can be caused if non-Hindus touch the body. Gloves should therefore be worn at all times. Relatives may wish to be informed of impending death to arrange performance of religious rituals. They may also wish to read from the Bhagavad-Gita. The family will usually want to care for the body (preferably at home), and the eldest son is required to remain present throughout. If the family is not available the following should be adhered to: Wearing gloves, close the eyes and mouth and straighten the limbs. Care should be taken not to remove any sacred threads, jewellery or ornamentation from the body. Wrap the body in a clean, plain sheet. Some relatives may request that the body be dressed in special clothing. Cleansing is done later as part of the funeral ritual. If the body is to be left overnight, a light or candle should be left burning throughout the night. If the family wish to view the deceased, care should be taken to ensure that the room is free of any other religious symbols or artefacts. The funeral is usually held within 24 hours. Post-mortem is considered disrespectful and will only be agreed to if required by law. Hindus will wish to be cremated.

Table 7.1 Last Offices: special considerations for different cultural and religious practices

Religion	Special considerations
Islam (Muslim)	Family members will wish to be present at death to perform last rites and will request that the client's head be pointed towards Mecca (south-east in the UK). Relatives or religious leaders usually perform Last Offices as soon as possible after death either at home or in the mosque. If there is no family present, staff wearing gloves should straighten the body, remove tubes, catheters, cannulae, etc., turn the head towards the right shoulder, facing Mecca, and cover the body with a clean white sheet. Under no circumstances should nails or hair be cut. Organ donation is only permitted with the express permission of the imam (religious leader) and post-mortem only agreed if required by law. Islam requires that the deceased be buried, preferably within 24 hours.
Jehovah's Witness	Relatives sometimes wish to stay during Last Offices to read prayers and will inform staff of any particular requests. The church does not object to post-mortem or organ donation; this is therefore a matter of individual choice. Both burial and cremation are acceptable.
Judaism	If at all possible a Jewish person or Holy Assembly should be present at death, and they will perform ritual prayer and washing. The body must be left for eight minutes immediately following death before it is touched, and the funeral must take place within 24 hours, though it cannot take place during the Sabbath (Friday sunset until Saturday sunset). If strict orthodox the body should be handled as little as possible. If handling by non-Jews is necessary, gloves must be worn. If relatives are not present staff should straighten the body with hands open and arms parallel and close to the body, close the mouth and eyes, and remove cannulae, drains, etc. The body should be dressed in a shroud and covered with a clean sheet. Relatives may request that the body be laid on the floor with the feet projecting towards the door. It is customary for someone to stay with the deceased from death until burial and prayers will be recited during this time.

Progressive Jews may be laid out as described in the text, while wearing gloves, but it is always advisable to check with the relatives or rabbi first if you are unsure. Post-mortem is only permitted if required by law. |
Mormon (Church of Jesus Christ of the Latter Day Saints)	Last Offices as outlined in the text are usually acceptable. Relatives may wish to remain present to recite prayers and to dress the deceased in sacred underwear. There are no religious objections to organ donation or post-mortem.
Rastafarian	Last Offices as outlined in the text are usually acceptable. Relatives may wish to remain present to recite prayers. Both post-mortem and organ donation are generally considered to be distasteful.
Sikhism	The family will wish to be present at death, particularly the eldest son, and will normally perform Last Offices. They may, however, ask staff to straighten the body, close the eyes and mouth, and cover the deceased with a clean sheet. Under no circumstances should the turban, shorts, wrist bracelet or sword be removed. Hair (including beard) and nails should not be cut, nor the 'Kanga' (comb) removed. Post-mortem is only permitted if required by law, and organ donation is not allowed.

Rationale

Performing Last Offices means 'caring for the body after death'. It is the final expression of caring a nurse can undertake for their client. It is also essential to maintaining a safe environment and ensuring safe passage of the body.

Equipment

Wash bowl

Soap and towel(s)

Disposable wipes

Shaving materials as required (electric shaving is preferable to avoid damage to the skin)

Toothbrush/toothpaste/oral hygiene pack

Brush/comb

Spigots and/or clamps (if necessary)

Adhesive tape

Occlusive tape and wound dressings if required

Disposable gloves and aprons

Clinical waste bag

Clean linen and laundry skip

Shroud or clean attire in keeping with deceased's/relatives' cultural/religious preferences

Property book and envelope for valuables

Legal documents; care records, medical notes, identification bands, death labels, notification-of-death forms

Body bag if required (see special precautions)

Procedure	Rationale
Screen the bed area, alert all members of staff including the senior nurse. Remove any unsightly clutter and unnecessary equipment and reassure other clients or staff who may be distressed	To maintain privacy and dignity for both client and relatives and to reduce the potential for further distress
Ensure that death has been verified by a doctor or senior nurse and that this has been documented in the client's records	To comply with legislation
Familiarize yourself with the client's/relatives' wishes and cultural and religious needs *before* touching the deceased, as procedures vary depending on religious beliefs (see Table 7.1)	Ensures respect for persons
Wear disposable aprons and other protective clothing as necessary (see 'Special precautions' below)	To reduce the likelihood of cross-infection

Procedure	Rationale
Lay the deceased in the supine position with arms by their sides and legs straight, and one pillow under the head (wear gloves if necessary to perform this task, in keeping with cultural/religious beliefs)	To maintain dignity, facilitate after-care and create an improved aesthetic look, should relatives wish to view the deceased following death
It is *not* recommended to place the hands under the body	Placing the hands under the body can cause bruising and discoloration
Remove all jewellery unless explicitly asked by relatives not to do so, document same and place in safekeeping following local policy	To adhere to legislative requirements and family's wishes
Provided that they are removed prior to 'viewing', a pillow may be placed under the jaw to close the mouth, and damp cotton wool or gauze may be rested on the eyelids	To assist closure
In some areas it is customary to leave the deceased in this position for one hour before commencing Last Offices	To allow the soul to depart
Provide the opportunity for the bereaved to view the deceased	To pay their last respects and assist grieving
Provide an environment conducive to viewing by: • ensuring privacy and dignity • removing dead/dying flowers and replacing with fresh ones if possible. Some health carers elect to place flowers on the body. Whilst this may be acceptable to some relatives it is not always welcomed, as some see this as the personal right of the next of kin. This practice is therefore not recommended unless you know the family well • covering the deceased with clean, fresh linen (some areas have dedicated linen such as a duvet or coloured counterpane) • ensuring lighting is subtle • controlling room temperature • ensuring good ventilation	Increases feelings of worth
• speaking quietly and avoiding unnecessary/inappropriate conversation in the vicinity of the bereaved	Reduces stress and anxiety
• offering to stay with the relatives if required • reducing environmental noise such as telephones, alarms, machinery, banging doors, and movement of equipment	Promotes psychological well-being and reduces fear and anxiety
• making sure there is adequate seating for the bereaved	To promote comfort

Procedure	Rationale
Determine that the family/religious leader have spent sufficient time with the deceased and reassure them that they can, if they wish, view the deceased in the chapel of rest later if they are not to be involved in the final acts	To allow grieving and completion of religious rituals
If relatives wish to remain to observe or participate in the remainder of the procedure, ensure at this juncture that they are fully conversant with what is to follow and clarify with them their intended degree of involvement and the point at which they would like to leave	To reduce the potential for added distress
Ensure that the family have details of what to do next, including: whether or not a post-mortem is necessary; where and when to collect the Medical Certificate of Death; what will happen to the deceased's belongings; and how to go about making funeral arrangements	To provide continuity of care
This information should be reinforced in writing; most clinical areas have preprinted booklets that can be given to relatives prior to their leaving. It is usual for the death to be registered in the town or city in which the death occurred. If the deceased or relatives are not local the death may be registered in the town or city where they lived; however, relatives need to be advised that this may lengthen the time it takes to arrange the funeral. The death must be registered within five days	Information retention is often severely limited in times of distress
Provide information about any support services available for the bereaved and advise that they may contact the clinical area for further guidance or information if they wish	To provide continuity of care
Ensure that the bereaved have some form of transport home	To demonstrate compassion and ensure safety
Ensure that you have all the necessary equipment to hand and advise other team members of your intentions	To prevent disturbances
Remove all hair clips and other metal objects as appropriate. If rings are to be left on the body these should be securely taped in position and documented on the death label (see Figure 7.2b). If the deceased has any internal metal devices, such as a pacemaker, these should also be clearly documented following local policy	To maintain safety of others

Procedure	Rationale
Remove any dressings, cannulae, etc. (unless a post-mortem is to be performed; see 'Special precautions' below). If there is any leakage from orifices or wounds these should be gently padded or packed and sealed with occlusive tape	To restore aesthetic state and reduce infection risk to others
If necessary express the bladder	To remove residual urine
Cleanse the body as necessary in keeping with the deceased's cultural/religious practices and dress the deceased in appropriate attire, such as shroud, nightdress or personal clothing	To restore aesthetic state. **NB** If the client's own clothes are used ensure that you have the express permission of the next of kin as it is unlikely that these will be removed prior to cremation/burial
Cleanse the mouth and return dentures if worn. If you experience difficulty in fitting the teeth these should be bagged and sent with the deceased to the mortuary and carefully documented	To restore aesthetic state and reduce infection risk to others
Leave the client's hospital identification bracelet in situ on the wrist (replace if illegible) and place similar on the client's opposite ankle in keeping with local policy. Death labels should be affixed to the body, usually one on the shroud over the deceased's chest, and one on the outer covering. The Death Notice (Figure 7.1) is usually placed with the body or client's records depending on local policy	To facilitate identification
Place a clean sheet under the client, leaving an adequate amount at each end to cover the head and feet. A 'sigh' may be heard when the deceased is rolled over as the residual air is expelled from the lungs. Some institutions also require the deceased to be placed on a canvas to facilitate moving and handling. Check local policy. If relatives are present they may wish to leave prior to the undertaking of the remainder of the procedure and should be given the opportunity to say their last farewells	To facilitate moving and handling
Tie the feet together if necessary	To keep the body in alignment
Wrap the sheet over the head and feet and then around the body, securing with adhesive tape	To avoid damage when transferring the deceased and to prevent distress to others
Clear away equipment and dispose of clinical waste appropriately. Remove gloves and apron and wash hands	Infection control

Procedure	Rationale
Complete the client's plan of care	To record time of death and surrounding circumstances
Contact portering services to remove the deceased from the clinical area following local policy	
Send property, suitably packed, and hospital records to the appropriate department and obtain signature for receipt of same. If any property is soiled, permission should be obtained from the relatives to dispose of same	To prevent any administrative incident which may cause additional distress
If it is the practice in your clinical area, screen remaining clients' bed areas when the portering staff come to collect the body	To reduce distress to others
Clean the bed following hospital policy and remake it before drawing back the curtains around the deceased's bed area	As above
Inform other clients and provide an opportunity to express their thoughts and feelings, as they are often very distressed by such an event	To allay fears, misconceptions and provide support
Both senior and less experienced staff often need further support and debriefing. Do not hesitate to share your feelings with your mentor or other members of the ward/department team. The chaplaincy can also be a useful source of support regardless of your religious or spiritual persuasion	To reduce distress

Special precautions

Clients receiving radiation therapy

The medical physics department should be informed immediately of the death so that they can make arrangements with the mortuary for removal of the body. The two members of staff undertaking Last Offices should wear gloves, aprons, gowns and plastic overshoes whilst performing this final act and they should endeavour to minimize, as much as is humanly possible, their contact with the body. All orifices should be carefully packed and any urine, blood or vomit must be cleared away. The body should be sealed in a plastic cadaver bag, and arrangements made by the medical physics department for removal of the body should be strictly adhered to.

Figure 7.1 Death notice

Hallam Lodge Hospital

Ward: ....

Copies to: Porters' Lodge
              Reception

Date: ....

Notification of Death

Re: ....

The above client died at ....am/pm on...20........

Next of kin...

*The relatives have been notified and were asked to attend

at.............................. on ....day

*The relatives have not yet been notified of the death

*Coroner's Case/P.M. requested

*Delete where applicable   .... Senior Nurse

Figure 7.2 Death label

a) Front

DEATH LABEL
PLEASE USE CAPITALS

Surname..Reg No..............
Forenames...
Address...
Age..............................Date of Death..............................
Consultant.............................Ward...................................

Details of property left on body to be recorded on reverse

b) Reverse side

Details of property left on body:

....

....

....

If no property, state "No Property".

Nurse's Signature ....

Witness ....

Clients who have or are suspected of having died with a Category 3 or 4 infectious disease

If the client has or is suspected of having a Category 3 or 4 infectious disease such as HIV, TB or hepatitis and thus a continued source of infection following death, then the body must be placed in a plastic cadaver bag and labelled appropriately, following local policy. This is not necessary for clients with MRSA.

Clients leaking body fluids

If the client is leaking body fluids and this cannot be stemmed with waterproof dressings or gentle packing, the body should be treated as above.

Clients requiring a post-mortem

These include all unexpected or unexplained deaths and any client dying within 24 hours of surgery. All drains, cannulae, tubes, etc. must be secured and left in situ. Spigots may be used as necessary to prevent leakage provided that care is taken not to dislodge them.

Other useful information

- It is increasingly common for clinical areas to set aside a specific room for bereaved relatives. If provided it is recommended that it be tastefully decorated, free from clutter and equipment, with comfortable seating and a telephone to facilitate communication with other family members and significant others.
- When preparing a client for viewing ensure that you remove all clutter such as excess pillows, linen, water jugs and any equipment no longer required. Be sure also to remove any flowers or plants that are clearly beyond their best.
- If the deceased is to donate organs, then the body should not be touched and the appropriate medical officer should be informed of the death immediately.
- The use of ring boxes to return jewellery can help minimize distress.
- If property is to be labelled 'DECEASED' this should be done subtly.
- Following the death, many relatives would welcome the opportunity to meet staff again, to thank them or ask questions. This desire can occur days, weeks or even months after the death. Relatives should therefore be made aware that this opportunity exists but that in order to ensure that they receive dedicated attention it would be best if they telephoned first to arrange a mutually convenient date and time.

- Some clinical areas keep a record of deaths and arrange to send a card or notelet on the first anniversary of the death. This is often greatly valued by the bereaved.
- Funeral arrangements can commence as soon as the relatives feel ready. It is not necessary to wait for the medical certificate. Relatives often ask about funeral directors; whilst it is not appropriate to make recommendations you can advise them that a list can be found in the local telephone directory or *Yellow Pages*.
- Those receiving income support, housing benefit or family credit may be able to get help with the cost of a funeral. Funeral directors can assist with making a claim.
- Relatives will need to telephone the registrar's office to arrange an appointment time. The person attending to register the death need not necessarily be the next of kin, although the individual will need the medical certificate from the hospital and be able to give the following personal details about the deceased:
  - the date and place of death
  - the deceased's full name, surname and maiden name if applicable
  - if the deceased was a married woman, the name and occupation of the husband
  - date and place of birth
  - the last occupation of the deceased
  - details of any state pension
  - date of birth of a surviving spouse
  - date of marriage
  - medical card or NHS number.
- Following registration the registrar issues two forms: one white, which should be sent to notify the Department of Social Security of the death along with any benefit books; and one green, which should be given to the funeral director along with the removal order issued by the hospital.
- The funeral director obtains the official forms necessary for burial or cremation once the death has been registered.
- Religious leaders can not only be a source of great comfort to the bereaved both initially and at a later stage, but they can also offer practical assistance in terms of funeral arrangements, memorial services and so on.
- A solicitor can assist with obtaining probate but this is not essential. Relatives can obtain probate personally by contacting the Probate Office and obtaining the necessary forms and direction.
- The Benefits Agency offers the useful booklet *What to do After a Death* on request.
- Banks, building societies, insurance companies, etc. often request a copy of the Registration of Death. Additional copies are best obtained when initially registering the death, as cost increases significantly if obtained at a later date.

If the body is to be sent abroad to the country of origin particular steps must be adhered to, but the funeral director or appointed religious leader will be fully conversant with these matters and usually manages this.

If you have any outstanding concerns or queries, further information can always be obtained from the hospital chaplaincy, which caters for all religious groups and denominations.

References and further reading

Akhtar S (2002) Nursing with dignity Part 8 - Islam. Nursing Times 98(16): 40-42.

Anonymous (2000) Essential Skills: 7 Last Offices: client hygiene. Nursing Standard 15(12) insert p2.

Baxter C (2002) Nursing with dignity Part 5 - Rastafarianism. Nursing Times 98(13): 42-43.

Becker R (1999) Teaching Communication with the dying across cultural boundaries. British Journal of Nursing 8(14): 938-42.

Black J (1987) Broaden your mind about death and bereavement in certain ethnic groups in Britain. British Medical Journal 295: 536-67.

Chauhan G, Long A (2000) Communication is the essence of nursing care 1: breaking bad news. British Journal of Nursing 9(14): 931-8.

Christmas M (2002) Nursing with dignity Part 3 - Christianity I. Nursing Times 98(11): 37-9.

Collins A (2002) Nursing with dignity Part 1 - Judaism. Nursing Times 98(9): 34-5.

Cowles KV (1996) Cultural perspective of grief: an expanded concept analysis. Journal of Advanced Nursing 23(2): 287-94.

Dickenson D, Johnson M, Katz JS (2000) Death, Dying and Bereavement. London: Sage.

Gill B (2002) Nursing with dignity Part 6 - Sikhism. Nursing Times 98(14): 39-41.

Green J (1991a) Death with Dignity: Meeting the Spiritual Needs of Clients in a Multi-cultural Society. London: Nursing Times/Macmillan Press.

Green J (1991b) Death with Dignity: Meeting the Spiritual Needs of Clients in a Multi-cultural Society, vol 2. London: Nursing Times/Macmillan Press.

Green J, Green M (1992) Dealing with Death - Practices and Procedures. London: Chapman Hall.

Jacob SR (1993) An analysis of the concept of grief. Journal of Advanced Nursing 18: 1787-94.

Jootun D (2002) Nursing with dignity Part 7 - Hinduism. Nursing Times 98(15): 38-40.

Kubler-Ross E (1990) Living with Dying and Death. London: Souvenir.

Mallett J, Dougherty L (2000) Royal Marsden Manual of Clinical Nursing Procedures, 5th edn. London: Blackwell Science.

Nearney L (2001) Practical Procedures for Nurses Series 14: Nursing Times. London: Emap Health Care.

Neuberger J (1994) Caring for Dying People of Different Faiths. London: Wolfe.

Northcott N (2002) Nursing with dignity Part 2 - Buddhism. Nursing Times 98(10): 36-8.

Nyatanga B (1997) Cultural issues in palliative care nursing. International Journal of Palliative Care 3(4): 203-208.

Papadopoulos I (2002) Nursing with dignity Part 4 - Christianity II. Nursing Times 98(12): 36-7.

Parkes CM, Laungani P, Young B (1997) Death and Bereavement Across Cultures. London: Routledge Press.

Roper N, Logan WW, Tierney A (1996) The Elements of Nursing. Edinburgh: Churchill Livingstone.

Royal College of Nursing (1981) Verification of Death and Performance of Last Offices. London: RCN.

Royal College of Pathologists (2000) Examination of the Body after Death. London: The Royal College of Pathologists, http://www.rcpath.org.

Sewell P (2002) Respecting a patient's care needs after death. Nursing Times 98(39): 36-7.

Simpson J (2002) Nursing with dignity Part 9 - Jehovah's Witnesses. Nursing Times 98(17): 36-7.

Speck P (1992) Care after death: the importance of Last Offices. Nursing Times 88(6): 20.

Chapter 8

Eliminating

Carol Pollard and Beverly Levy

Introduction

The act of elimination is a fundamental human process essential to life. Being able to meet clients' elimination needs is therefore an essential nursing function and can help to both maintain and/or restore a client's well-being and preserve life. The skills involved do, however, need to be applied sensitively, as many clients despair at the thought of being unable to manage their own toilet requirements. Remember, many of the nursing interventions required are of a very intimate nature, for example cleansing the perineum following defecation or dealing with a client's menstrual flow. Gaining the client's trust and confidence, along with their permission, is therefore crucial. Bladder and bowel care forms one of the first wave of topics covered in the Department of Health's document *Essence of Care* in which they outline 11 benchmarks for best practice. These can be found at http://www.doh.gov.uk/essenceofcare. Following is a brief introduction to the processes of elimination.

Elimination of urine

The urinary system is an excretory system of the body and consists of a number of structures. We have two kidneys responsible for water and electrolyte balance and the formation of urine by simple filtration, selective reabsorption and secretion. They secrete urine at approximately 1 ml per minute provided the individual is adequately hydrated. We also have two ureters, responsible for carrying the urine from the kidneys to the urinary bladder by peristaltic contraction of their muscle walls; and one urinary bladder, which acts as a reservoir where urine is stored prior to being excreted. Finally, we have one urethra, a channel leading from the bladder through which urine is excreted. In females this is quite short, measuring about 3.6 cm in an adult, whereas in males it has to extend the length of the penis and is therefore between 20 and 22.5 cm in a mature adult.

Elimination of faecal waste

The waste products of digestion are excreted through the bowel. They pass from the ileum through the ileo-caecal valve into the caecum. In the large intestine absorption of water occurs until the semi-solid consistency of faeces is achieved. Mass movement forces the contents of the pelvic colon into the rectum where the nerve endings in its wall are stimulated by stretching. When the stretch receptors in the rectum are stimulated beyond a certain point nerve impulses are conveyed to the consciousness, telling us that our bowel needs emptying, though the brain can normally help us inhibit the reflex until such a time that it is convenient to defecate. The frequency of need to empty the bowel can vary markedly between individuals; some people may normally expect a movement daily whilst others might only pass a motion once every two to three days.

Whilst the urinary system and bowel function independently of one another both need to function efficiently in order to excrete body waste effectively. Excretion of waste products is essential to maintaining health and well-being. Inadequate bladder and bowel function can ultimately affect homeostasis (that is, the body's delicate fluid, electrolyte and acid–base balance) and lead to serious illness and even death.

Elimination of menstrual waste

Procreation, or the ability to produce offspring, is an essential function of living beings if they are to remain a viable species. Reproduction is dependent on the female producing ova (eggs) for the male to fertilize with sperm. The production and release of the eggs occurs in monthly cycles, which commence around the age of 11–13 years and cease when the woman reaches the menopause, most frequently around the age of 50. The secretion of the hormones oestrogen and progesterone influences this cycle, though a number of other factors, such as diet, stress, medication and contraceptive devices, can also influence an individual's pattern.

The female reproductive system consists of two ovaries, responsible for releasing the eggs, and two Fallopian tubes that carry the eggs to the uterus. The uterus is a hollow, pear-shaped muscular organ, which retains the egg prior to fertilization.

Uterine and ovarian cycles are usually referred to as the menstrual cycle. The first day of bleeding in a non-pregnant, fertile woman, when blood, secretions and the top layer of the endometrium is shed, is generally considered day 1 of the cycle. The menstrual cycle usually lasts about 28 days, but bleeding only occurs for 4–5 of these days. Ovulation, when the egg or ovum is released from the ovary, usually occurs on or about day 14.

The factors that affect elimination may be:

- ...sing from alteration in the structure, function or processes of gastro-intestinal or associated bodily systems
- ...*al* such as intellect, anxiety and stress
- ...*al*, for example different words used for elimination and products ...on, different rituals surrounding elimination (such as clean hand ...ng, dirty hand for cleansing), fasting and other dietary restrictions
- ...*vironmental* including poor food storage, personal hygiene and toileting facilities
- *politico-economic*, for example lack of finances for a healthy high-fibre diet, political influences on availability of certain foods and genetically modified products.

The remainder of this chapter gives the common terminology associated with the activity of eliminating; points to consider when assessing an individual's ability to eliminate; how to assist clients to eliminate; how to apply a nappy; care of an indwelling urinary catheter; monitoring urinary output; bowel actions and vomit; and how to collect specimens of urine and faeces. The chapter concludes with references and further reading.

Common terminology

Alkaptonuria	A rare hereditary disorder characterized by excessive secretion of homogentistic acid in the urine
Anuria	Absence of or failure to produce urine
Catheter	A slender, hollow tube of varying lengths, bores (diameters) and shapes that is inserted into a bodily structure; in the case of a urinary catheter the structure is the bladder
Constipation	Infrequent and often difficult evacuation of faeces or the passage of hard stools less frequently than the client's own normal pattern
Continence	The ability to retain bodily excrement, that is, urine and faeces, until such time as is appropriate to eliminate them
Cystitis	Inflammation of the bladder
Diaphoresis	Perspiration, particularly if excessive
Defecation	The discharge of waste products from the rectum
Diarrhoea	Loose and sometimes watery, frequent evacuation of stools, with or without discomfort
Dysuria	Difficulty passing urine
Eclampsia	A severe form of toxaemia, which occurs in pregnancy and can lead to convulsions, coma and death

Frequency	The felt need to pass urine more often than normal
Haemorrhoids	Protruding vein in the rectal area
Homeostasis	The automated self-regulation of humans to maintain the normal state of the body under a variety of conditions
Incontinence	Inability to resist the urge to urinate or defecate
Indole	A product of intestinal putrefaction
Meatus	The external opening of the urethra
Meleana	Black, tarry stools as a result of digesting blood
Menstruation	The periodic shedding of blood, secretions and cells from the uterus of a non-pregnant, fertile woman, lasting 4–5 days, this usually occurs in cycles of approximately 28 days and is influenced by the excretion of oestrogen and progesterone
Micturition	The act of passing urine
Motion	A term sometimes used for a bowel movement
Myoglobin	Muscle protein that transports oxygen
Nocturia	Excessive passing of urine in the night
Skatole	A strong-smelling nitrogen compound in human faeces
Steatorrhoea	Pale, bulky, fatty stools
Stoma	An artificial opening established surgically between an organ and the exterior
Stool	Another term sometimes used for a bowel movement
Suprapubic	Situated above the pubic bone
Urethritis	Inflammation of the urethra
Urgency	A sudden strong desire to pass urine
Urinate	To discharge urine from the body
Voiding urine	Emptying the bladder

Assessing the individual's ability to eliminate

Obtaining an assessment of a client's elimination pattern can be quite a challenge. The client may feel very uncomfortable with the idea of talking about this subject, and differences in the use of words to refer to a wish to pass urine or defecate can mean that information is misinterpreted. Issues surrounding menstruation are also generally considered private. The nurse therefore needs to be sensitive to these issues during the assessment of this activity of living. As with other aspects of assessment a private room, away from other people, is the ideal place to undertake exploration of a client's elimination patterns and needs. Whilst such a venue is often difficult to find on a busy ward, a setting that provides as much privacy as possible should be sought to promote client comfort when talking to the health care professional.

When eliciting information about the clients' normal elimination patterns, this information needs to be specific so you should avoid using vague words such as 'regular' without clarifying the meaning with the client.

Remember that assessment of elimination is only part of a holistic nursing assessment and should not be undertaken in isolation without reference to or consideration of the client's other activities of living.

Specific points to consider when assessing an individual's ability to eliminate are:

- *Physical*
  How often do they pass urine?
  Do they have to get up in the night to pass urine; if so how often?
  How often do they have a bowel movement? Is this their norm?
  Would they say they were constipated?
  Do they have diarrhoea?
  What colour is the faeces? Is there any blood, fat or mucus present?
  Does the faeces float?
  Do they experience any pain/burning when passing urine or faeces?
  Does their urine smell or is it offensive?
  Does their faeces smell more offensively than normal?
  Does the client experience any other difficulties when attempting to pass urine or faeces, for example frequency, urgency, difficulty initiating flow?
  Have they noticed any other significant changes in their elimination habits?
  Are they taking any medication that might affect elimination, for example codeine compounds?
  Are they receiving adequate dietary and fluid intake to promote normal functioning?
  Any evidence of incontinence, dribbling, retention?
  Does the client have any changes in mode of elimination such as a stoma or catheter?
  Are there any other factors that may influence their ability to eliminate, for example reduced mobility?
  What is the client's usual menstrual cycle and where are they in that cycle (if X-rays are to be undertaken)?
  Is bleeding generally normal/heavy/light/painful?
  Does the client get particularly emotional at this time?
  Does the client take any medication that is prescribed for or that might affect their elimination patterns, for example laxatives, water tablets, HRT, contraception?

- *Psychological*
  Is the client anxious, depressed, worried or frightened?
  Are they embarrassed?

Does the client require any toilet training or assistance in re-establishing elimination patterns?

- *Sociocultural*
  Does the client follow any particular religious, social or cultural rituals associated with elimination?
  Does the client use any particular words or phrases for urine, faeces, defecation, etc.?
  Does the client have an established hygiene ritual following toileting?
  Does the client take regular exercise? Reduced mobility can lead to constipation.

- *Environmental*
  Do they have access to toilet facilities?
  Are these satisfactory and/or appropriate?
  Do they have any adequate facilities for storing, cooking and handling food?
  Do they have any educational needs in relation to food storage, cooking and handling?
  Does the client have adequate equipment to meet their hygiene needs in relation to their menstrual cycle?
  Do they know where to dispose of tampons/sanitary towels, etc.?

- *Politico-economic*
  Does the client have adequate finances for a healthy, well-balanced diet?
  Has the increasing closure of public toilet facilities impacted on the client in any way?
  Do they have adequate funds for menstrual protection?

Assisting clients to use toileting facilities

Nurses and carers, in partnership with the client, need to assess the most appropriate vessel for the client to eliminate into based on their current situation.

Using the toilet

Ideally, individuals prefer to use the toilet, as from a very early age we are taught that this is the most appropriate place to eliminate. Therefore if a person can maintain this normality despite illness or disability it should be encouraged and supported, to promote psychological well-being. This can simply involve the nurse or other health care professional helping the client to locate the whereabouts of the toilet if they are in a new environment.

Adaptations can be made to the toilet if required to enable a person to continue to use the toilet if, due to mobility problems, this is becoming difficult. Raised toilet seats and rails can help some people to get on and off the toilet and help them to continue to meet their elimination needs independently.

Using a commode

If a person is unable to get to the toilet then a commode can be used. The nurse can either wheel the client to the toilet on the commode, or the client can use the commode at the side of their bed.

When a person is using a commode the nurse or other carer needs to ensure that the commode is cleaned before and after use. Washing with soap and water is usually perfectly adequate provided that it is subsequently dried. If the client is safe to be left alone while they are on the commode/toilet the nurse must ensure that they have easy access to the nurse call system so they can get the assistance quickly when they have finished. Numerous complaints made by clients and their relatives identify that some clients have been left for long periods of time in a toilet or on a commode before a nurse has returned to help them. This is a very frightening experience for the client, as well as uncomfortable and potentially dangerous.

Using a bedpan or urinal

If a client is unable to go to the toilet then a bedpan or urinal will be required.

When assisting a client with their elimination needs, standard precautions should be applied. You should wear a plastic apron and gloves if you are likely to come into contact with body fluids. Hand hygiene following these activities is essential to reduce the risk of cross-infection. The client's hygiene needs should also be considered. Providing the client with time and the facilities to wash their own hands after going to the toilet is essential. The client may also require assistance to wash their perineal area.

Most bedpans and urinals in institutional settings are now disposable and can be discarded in the macerator. If caring for a client in an alternative environment, however, it may well be that you will need to dispose of the contents down the toilet and then wash the receptacle in hot soapy water before returning it to the client. Take care of course to accurately record any output if required.

In the case of disposable urinals, it is usually desirable for both the client and the carer to leave them with a replacement. This not only serves to increase the individual's autonomy but also means that they do not get upset about having to ask, and that they do not have to wait next time should you be busy.

Applying/changing a nappy

Rationale

To maintain personal hygiene and comfort, to monitor urinary and faecal output and to assess and/or maintain skin integrity.

Equipment

Changing mat
Clean disposable nappy or cotton nappy, liner and safety pin(s)
Clean clothing/bedding as required
Bowl, water and soap or cleansing wipes
Barrier cream

Procedure	Rationale
Wash and dry hands thoroughly and don gloves and apron	To prevent cross-infection
Assess the infant's nappy for soiling and wetness	To determine equipment needs
Determine the infant's stage of development	To determine care needs
Assess the type and size of nappy required	To ensure correct fit
Collect and prepare equipment and environment	To promote infant safety
Place the infant on a flat surface and keep at least one hand on the infant at all times	To prevent the infant falling. **NB** Never leave an infant unattended either out of the cot or in a cot with the side down
Remove the soiled nappy noting colour, amount and consistency of any faecal material	To aid evaluation and future care planning. **NB** In critical-care areas it may be necessary to weigh the nappy to ensure

Procedure	Rationale
	accurate monitoring of input and output. This is achieved by comparing the weight of a clean nappy with the soiled nappy. One millilitre is approximately = one gramme. If in doubt, always check before disposing of the nappy and its contents
Roll the nappy to retain the contents and place out of reach of the infant	To maintain safety
Clean the genitalia, groin and perineum (from front to back for females and the tip of the penis to the scrotum for males) with warm water and wipes	To restore hygiene and reduce the potential for soreness and cross-infection. Cotton wool should not be used as fibres may be left on the skin
Commercially produced baby wipes may be used once the infant reaches two weeks of age	Commercially produced baby wipes are not recommended for babies under two weeks of age as they destroy the normal skin flora
Assess skin integrity noting any redness, swelling, marks, allergy or other disorders of integrity and treat as appropriate	To identify actual/potential problems and initiate care. If in doubt about appropriate care needs seek guidance from a more experienced member of staff
If the skin is sore and reddened, a barrier cream should be applied	Barrier cream prevents urine and faeces coming into contact with the skin and allows it to heal
With one hand lift the infant's buttocks and with the other place the clean nappy underneath (thickest part forwards)	For ease of application and to maintain infant safety
Pull the front of the nappy through the legs and ensure a snug, but not tight, fit round the legs and waist (below the umbilical cord if this is still healing) and secure with tapes or safety pin as appropriate	To prevent the nappy falling off whilst reducing the potential for pressure sore development. **NB** If safety pins are used you should place your fingers between the nappy and the infant and insert from front to back to prevent injury
Change other clothing/bedding if soiled	To maintain hygiene and skin integrity
Return the infant to his/her cot and secure cot sides before leaving infant	To ensure infant safety
Dispose of equipment and soiled materials following local policies, and wash hands	To prevent cross-infection

Procedure	Rationale
Document output on fluid balance record/ stool chart. Report any abnormalities in evaluation and either modify care plan accordingly or alert a more senior member of staff	Legal requirement to maintain documentation and safeguard infant through effective communication

Care of an indwelling urinary catheter

A urinary catheter is a hollow tube that is inserted into the bladder to drain urine. They can be used intermittently, short term or long term. However, insertion of a urinary catheter should only ever be performed if sound justification can be advanced, as the risk of infection both during and following insertion is very high and can lead to prolonged hospitalization and even death in susceptible individuals.

Given the inherent risk of developing a urinary tract infection following catheterization it is vital that a health care professional explain to the client how to care for their catheter. If the client is unable to care for the catheter then the nurse or carer should be able to competently carry out the following procedures in keeping with local policy.

Emptying a catheter bag

If a catheter is left in the bladder to drain urine continuously, the urine will pass through a closed circuit and be stored in a sterile drainage bag until the client or nurse empties it.

Equipment

> Gloves
> Apron
> Clean measuring jug
> Chlorhexidine or other wipes (see local policy)
> Paper towel

Each time a catheter bag is emptied the closed system is disrupted. The more times this is done, the greater the risk of infection. The bag should therefore only be emptied when necessary, to reduce this risk. However, if the catheter bags are allowed to fill to capacity they can become very heavy and increase the drag factor for the client – that is, the pressure on the bladder neck should the bag inadvertently be dropped or allowed to pull. The interval between emptying a catheter bag therefore needs to be assessed on an individual basis.

Procedure	Rationale
Explain the procedure to the client	To obtain consent, gain co-operation and teach the client how to do this themselves if able
Wash hands, put on gloves and cover clothing with plastic apron	To minimize the risk of cross-infection
Clean the outlet portal according to local policy and allow to dry	To minimize the risk of cross-infection
Place the measuring jug below the outlet and release the tap	To prevent spillage
Once all the urine has drained, dry the outlet, wipe with a clean wipe and cover the container with the paper towel	To minimize infection risk
Remove to sluice and observe drainage. Note colour, smell, etc. as detailed in section 'Monitoring urinary output' below; measure the amount if required; and then dispose of the contents in the sluice or toilet	To monitor output and reduce the risk of contamination
Remove gloves and apron, and wash hands	To minimize the risk of cross-infection
Record findings in client's care records as appropriate and report any abnormalities	To maintain records, facilitate good communications and ensure that the client receives any necessary care and treatment

Cleaning the catheter and surrounding area

To reduce the risk of infection, the area of the client's body around the catheter should be washed with soap and water at least twice a day and following a bowel action. Clients with an indwelling catheter should be encouraged to perform this activity as part of their normal hygiene routine.

Procedure	Rationale
Explain the procedure to the client	To obtain consent and gain co-operation
Prepare equipment, bowel, warm water, cloth, soap, wipes and disposal receptacle	To ensure that everything required is available
Wash hands and put on gloves	To minimize the risk of contamination
Using a cloth/wipe, soap and water, swab away from the urethral opening	To reduce the risk of ascending infection
Ensure that the client is comfortable	To maintain quality nursing practice
Remove gloves and wash hands	To minimize the risk of cross-infection
Report any purulent discharge from around the catheter	To enable action to be taken and to increase the frequency of cleansing

Removing a urinary catheter

To restore client comfort and promote normal functioning.

Equipment

Apron
Gloves
Receiver
Syringe
Disposal receptacle

Procedure	Rationale
Explain the procedure to the client	To obtain consent and gain co-operation
Check the client's records for the volume of water in the balloon and ensure that the amount inserted is that of the volume removed	To prevent trauma to the urethra
Assist the client into the supine position (see Chapter 2)	This position provides maximum access
Place a receiver between the client's legs	To catch urine and prevent any spillage onto the bed

Procedure	Rationale
Wash hands and put on gloves	To reduce the risk of contamination
If necessary clean the area of the client's body around the catheter using soap and water	To minimize the risk of contamination during removal
Change gloves	Gloves have become contaminated during the cleaning of the meatus
Deflate the balloon using a syringe to remove the water	
Explain to the client that discomfort may be felt as the catheter is removed	To keep client informed and to gain co-operation
Ask the client to relax, then gently and smoothly remove the catheter	To reduce discomfort to the client
Clean the meatus and make the client comfortable	To reduce the risk of infection
Remove gloves, dispose of equipment and wash hands	To reduce the risk of cross-infection
Document the date and time of catheter removal	To maintain nursing records and continuity of care
Record the subsequent urine output and record on a fluid balance chart until frequency and amount is within normal limits. Observe for difficulty in voiding urine	To enable action to be taken promptly if any difficulties occur
Encourage the client to drink at least 2-3 litres of oral fluids daily (if allowed)	To promote production of urine

Monitoring urinary output

Normal urinary output is approximately 1.5 litres in 24 hours and the usual frequency of micturition is between 5 and 10 times in that period. However, this can be influenced significantly by the amount of fluid a person drinks and how much fluid they are losing through sweating, mental state and lifestyle.

Urine normally consists of:

96%	water
2%	urea
2%	uric acid, creatinine, sodium, potassium, chlorides, phosphates, sulphates, oxalates.

These are all waste products of the body's utilization of food and fluid.

The intensity of colour of normal urine depends on the concentration, and usually ranges from yellow to amber. Fresh urine does not have a strong odour and it should be clear when voided.

When monitoring a client's urine, important clues can be gained simply by careful observation. For example, greenish or yellow-brown urine could contain bile pigments and may indicate problems with liver function, whilst blood and haemoglobin will give a red-brown colour if present in quite large quantities. Some drugs, foods and dyes may also change the colour of urine. If any abnormalities are found they should be documented, reported and further investigations undertaken in consultation with the medical staff. If you suspect that blood is present in the urine, and if the client is female, check whether or not they are menstruating before reporting, as menstrual blood can give a false positive result.

Measuring urine output

If it is necessary to monitor the quantity and frequency of urine this should be recorded on the client's fluid balance chart as given in Figure 5.5.

If a client's urine output is to be measured the procedure is as given below.

Procedure	Rationale
Explain why and how the urine will be collected and measured	To gain the client's consent and co-operation
Provide the client with a bedpan or urinal when they want to pass urine	So that urine can be collected
Wash hands, wear plastic apron and gloves when collecting and measuring urine	To prevent contamination with body fluids
Empty the urine from the bedpan into a measuring jug taking care not to splash your face. If this is a potential risk in your area of care it is best to wear goggles to protect your eyes	To gain an accurate measure of the urine output. This activity should always be undertaken in the sluice, dirty utility area or toilet to minimize the risk of spreading infection

Procedure	Rationale
Note amount	
Dispose of the urine in the macerator, sluice or toilet, rinse the measuring jug and store dry	To reduce the risk of cross-infection
Remove gloves and apron and dispose in keeping with local policy	To reduce the risk of cross-infection
Wash and dry hands thoroughly	To reduce the risk of cross-infection
Accurately record urine output on fluid balance chart	To monitor fluid balance and plan care accordingly
For an infant or child see section on 'Applying/changing a nappy'	

Performing urinalysis

Urinalysis, or analysis of urine, is important as disturbances of normal physiological functions are often reflected in the urine. Analysis of the urine can provide important clues as to what is going on elsewhere in the body and thus aid diagnosis. It can also assist in monitoring the disease process and efficacy of treatment.

Equipment

> Clean container
> Reagent strips
> Apron
> Gloves
> Appropriate documentation

Procedure	Rationale
Explain the procedure to the client	To gain co-operation and ensure understanding
Provide an environment conducive to the task; that is, one that offers visual and auditory privacy	To avoid embarrassment and maintain privacy and dignity
Ask the client to void into a clean container. Disposable containers are ideal	To minimize bacterial and chemical contamination

Procedure	Rationale
For infants and small children, specifically designed containers are obtained which adhere to the perineum. Care should be taken to follow the manufacturer's instructions when applying and removing these so that the child's skin integrity is not broken	To facilitate collection of specimen. A child's skin is very delicate and can easily be damaged
Observe the specimen for colour and odour	To identify any possible abnormalities
Check that the reagent strips have not expired and that they have been stored according to the manufacturer's instructions	To reduce the potential for inaccurate results. **NB** Manufacturers always supply detailed instructions with the reagent strips and these should always be adhered to; however, some general principles apply: • Strips should always be stored in the bottle supplied and never decanted, to avoid contamination • The bottle cap should be replaced securely immediately after removing a strip for use, and the desiccant should never be removed from the bottle as the strips can become damp • The bottle should be stored in a cool dry place but not refrigerated, for optimum results • Strips should not be used after the expiry date on the bottle
Dip the test strip into the urine ensuring that you wet the entire test pad	To facilitate accurate results
Withdraw the strip and tap gently on the rim of the container to remove any excess urine	To enable accurate reading and reduce the risk of contamination of self
Compare the colour of each test pad with those on the label of the container at the times indicated by the manufacturer, noting any abnormalities and making sure that you do not contaminate the container with urine	To ensure accurate results. Contaminated containers must be discarded to avoid cross-infection
Record results in nursing records and report any abnormalities (see Table 8.1)	To provide a record, facilitate good communications and ensure that the client receives any necessary care and treatment

Table 8.1 Urinalysis findings

Substance	Indication
Protein	A morning specimen is best for detecting abnormal levels of protein, which may indicate hypertension, pre-eclampsia, glomerulonephritis, infection or diabetes mellitus. Normal urine has a low level of albumen.
Blood	The presence of blood can indicate infection, renal stones, malignancy or injury to the urinary tract or kidneys. Blood is not normally present in urine; however, a false positive result can sometimes be obtained during menstruation. If an infection is suspected, the client should be asked if they have symptoms such as urgency, frequency, or pain or burning on micturition.
Ketones	Produced by the breakdown of fatty acids. Can be indicative of poorly controlled diabetes mellitus, dieting or anorexia.
Nirate	Optimal results are obtained from first morning specimen of urine, or urine passed four hours after the last voiding. Not normally present in urine, it is indicative of infection.
Glucose	Present if renal absorption is impaired, or if the client has raised blood glucose levels. Not normally present in urine.
Urobilinogen	Small amount normally present, but elevated levels indicate hepatic abnormalities or red blood cell breakdown.
Bilirubin	May indicate biliary disease. In conjunction with raised levels of urobilinogen it may indicate hepatic disease.
Leucocytes	A presence of leucocytes suggests an infection in the urinary tract.
pH	A pH greater than 7 may indicate infection. A strongly acidic pH may indicate fever, gout or metabolic acidosis. The average urine is slightly acidic and usually is within a pH of 5-6 but can vary with dietary intake from 4.8 to 8.5. Values are usually lowest after an overnight fast and highest after meals. Urine pH can be a helpful screening test in the diagnosis of renal, respiratory and certain metabolic diseases, and some treatment regimens such as sodium bicarbonate.
Specific gravity	This monitors the concentration and diluting power of the kidneys and assists in interpretation of other tests. Measuring specific gravity (SG) is a quick, convenient and reliable test for doing this. It is particularly valuable in helping us recognize dehydration. Normal SG is usually somewhere in the region of 1.000-1.030.

Appearance of the urine

Urine is usually clear but may vary from straw colour to darkish yellow or orange. Uncharacteristic colours are due to a variety of naturally occurring pigments from endogenous substances or various exogenous chemicals.

- Cloudy urine may indicate infection and is caused by the presence of particles that settle as sediment when urine is left to stand.
- A milky appearance may indicate contamination with chyle, spermatozoa, or acid or alkaline urine.
- A blue/green colour may indicate *Pseudomonas* infection or the presence of bilirubin. It can also be caused by methylene blue, a dye used in the manufacture of some medicines such as 'liver pills'.
- A pink/red colour may indicate the presence of blood, though some drugs or ingestion of certain foods such as beetroot can also produce this colour in the urine.
- An orange colour usually indicates particular drugs including rifampicin and some laxatives. It can also indicate the presence of urobiligen.
- A yellow colour may indicate conjugated bilirubin.
- A brown colour may indicate bilirubin or clients taking L-dopa.
- Brown/black urine may indicate alkaptonuria or the presence of myoglobin if the colour develops after the urine has been standing.

Odour

Fresh urine has very little smell, but will begin to smell of ammonia if left to stand.

- Infected urine has a foul, fishy smell.
- The sweet smell of acetone (pear drops or nail varnish remover) indicates the presence of ketones.
- Eating fish, curry or other strongly flavoured foodstuff can also make the urine smell.
- Certain medications, such as menthol antibiotics, and some vitamins can also affect the odour of urine.

If any abnormality is suspected it is usual to obtain a specimen of urine.

Collection of a specimen of urine

Observing and testing a specimen of a person's urine can tell us a great deal about their general health. Following routine urinalysis it may be necessary to obtain a specimen to send to the laboratory for further, more in-depth analysis. In doing so there are some general principles to be considered:

- Urine specimens should be tested as soon after collection as possible. Consequently if specimens cannot be transported to the laboratory and examined within two hours of collection they must be stored in an appropriate refrigeration unit at 4°C. However, they should not be stored for longer than 24 hours otherwise any findings will be inaccurate.

- Assessment of the client's physical and mental capacity prior to collecting a specimen of urine is essential in order to ensure that they can comply with the needs of the procedure, particularly if a mid-stream specimen (MSU) or a 24-hr collection is required. For an MSU, the client must urinate in the toilet or other receptacle, stop, pass urine into the specimen container or sterile receptacle, stop and then finish urinating as normal. If you wish to collect all the urine that the client passes in a 24-hr period (24-hr urine collection), special bottles containing preservatives and other chemicals are usually obtainable from the laboratory.

- For some investigations an early morning specimen may be required (EMU). It is therefore important to check the request form prior to undertaking the procedure, to ensure that the correct type of specimen is obtained.

Collecting a mid-stream specimen (MSU)

Procedure	Rationale
Explain the procedure to the client	To gain consent from the client and assess the amount of assistance they will require
Collect sterile specimen bottle, cleaning equipment and bedpan or urinal if required	To ensure that the specimen is not contaminated and to ensure that all equipment is to hand
Wash hands and apply gloves and plastic apron	To minimize risk of contamination
Wash client's perineal area with soap and water and pat dry	To minimize micro-organisms contaminating sample
Clean meatus with antiseptic solution and allow to dry	To reduce risk of contamination
Ask client to commence voiding into bedpan/urinal/toilet	Flushes organisms from urethral opening
Place specimen bottle under stream of urine	To collect specimen of urine that is least likely to be contaminated

Procedure	Rationale
Remove specimen bottle and allow client to continue to empty bladder	Prevents end-of-stream organisms dropping into specimen bottle
For infants and small children, specifically designed containers are obtained which adhere to the perineum. Care should be taken to follow the manufacturer's instructions when applying and removing these so that the child's skin integrity is not broken	To facilitate collection of specimen. A child's skin is very delicate and can easily be damaged
Remove gloves and plastic apron and wash hands	Minimizes risk of cross-infection
Ensure specimen is correctly labelled, and placed in appropriate plastic bag for transportation accompanied by request form	To prevent misidentification. To minimize risk to others
Dispatch the specimen to the laboratory immediately	To ensure validity of test

Collecting a catheter specimen of urine

A catheter specimen of urine is taken for bacteriological examination when there are symptoms of a urinary tract infection. It is an aseptic technique, to reduce the risk of contaminating the sample. Urine should be obtained from a specific port on the drainage bag – never by disconnecting the closed circuit. Nurses need to familiarize themselves with the sampling ports on the drainage ports.

Equipment

> 20 ml syringe
> 21G needle
> Universal container
> Gate clamp
> Microbiology form
> Alcohol swabs
> Receiver
> Gloves
> Apron
> Sharps box

Procedure	Rationale
Explain to the client why the specimen is required, and provide privacy	To gain co-operation, obtain consent and respect dignity
Clamp the drainage tubing just below the sampling port until sufficient urine is collected	To achieve sufficient urine for analysis
Never clamp the catheter	May damage the catheter
Collect equipment	Organization of equipment helps the procedure to run smoothly
Wash hands and put on gloves	To minimize the risk of contamination
Swab the sample port with a 70 per cent alcohol swab and allow the port to dry	To reduce the risk of infection
Insert the needle into the port at an angle of 45 degrees	To avoid going straight through the tube and therefore increasing the risk of needlestick injury
If no needle is required, insert the syringe firmly into the centre of the sample port and continue	Follows recommendations of manufacturer
Withdraw the required amount of urine. Remove the needle from the port. Remove the top of the specimen pot and fill it with urine	To obtain specimen
Dispose of needle and syringe immediately in a sharps box	To reduce the risk of needlestick injury
Swab the sample port with a 70 per cent alcohol swab and allow the port to dry	To reduce the risk of infection
Unclamp the catheter, remove gloves and dispose of equipment safely. Wash hands and make the client comfortable	To reduce the risk of injury and infection
Label the specimen container and transfer it to the laboratory with the request form	For identification of the client
Specimens should be transferred within one hour of sampling whenever possible	If transfer is delayed then specimens should be stored in a refrigerator at 4ºC. Storing them at room temperature for longer than two hours will affect the result
Document in the client's nursing records the date and time that the specimen was collected	To communicate this information to others

Monitoring bowel actions

Bowel habits are variable between individuals and are influenced by lifestyle, eating habits and mental state. The average adult will pass 100–150 g of faeces once per day; change in this pattern and change in the nature of faeces passed can indicate disease. The health care professional will therefore need to monitor the bowel action of clients where actual or potential problems are indicated.

Normal faeces is made up of 75 per cent water and 25 per cent solid constituents (cellulose, dead epithelial cells, bacteria, mucus and bile pigments). Skatole and indole arise from bacterial decomposition and give faeces it characteristic odour. Faecal matter is normally brown in colour, soft in consistency and cylindrical in form.

The carer should observe the client's faeces to identify any changes, and this should be documented in the client's records or on a stool chart along with frequency of passage and appearance of the faeces. The Bristol Stool Chart is a useful classification system that has been developed to assist us in recording the stool type and can be found on the Internet (www.bolton.nhs.uk/services/continence). This information can assist in diagnosis and treatment and can inform care planning.

Constipation is the commonest problem that can occur. This is the passage of hard stools less frequently than the client's normal pattern. Conversely, the term diarrhoea is used when faeces contains excess water and the frequency of defecation is markedly increased. Alternating constipation and diarrhoea is suggestive of irritable bowel syndrome but can indicate a partial obstruction.

Other less common abnormalities are:

- pale, putty-coloured faeces, indicative of problems in the biliary system
- presence of pus or excessive mucus, suggesting infection or inflammation
- black and tarry stools (meleana) with a characteristic smell of altered blood, suggestive of bleeding somewhere in the large bowel
- fresh blood in the faeces, which can indicate haemorrhoids or other abnormality
- black stools also occur as a result of taking iron tablets
- parasites
- foreign bodies, particularly in children, who may for example have swallowed a coin or placed something in their rectum.

All of these abnormalities usually require further investigation; therefore, a faecal specimen will be required.

Collection of specimen of faeces

Any persistent alteration in a client's bowel habits needs to be investigated as it may indicate a serious disorder. Therefore, the nurse may be required to collect a specimen of faeces, which will be sent to the laboratory for investigation. Single specimens may be collected for microscopy, culture and sensitivity if an infection is suspected, to determine the micro-organisms. Three consecutive specimens may be requested if we are looking for blood not detectable by the human eye (faeces for occult blood, FOB) or, if the client is passing pale, bulky stools, we sometimes collect *all* faecal output for three consecutive days (faecal fat collection). It is therefore important to ascertain which type of specimen is required and assess the client's ability to co-operate beforehand.

Equipment

> Bedpan (and sundries as necessary)
> Appropriate specimen container duly labelled with client's details, date and
>   accurate time of collection
> Completed specimen forms
> Plastic bag
> Category-3 stickers if client is considered a high risk
> Gloves

Procedure	Rationale
Explain the procedure to the client and ensure understanding and ability to participate, as necessary	To gain the client's consent and co-operation
Provide client with a clean bedpan	To reduce the risk of contaminating the specimen
Place the bedpan on the toilet/ commode	To ensure privacy for the client
Wash hands and put on gloves and disposable apron before handling the bedpan containing the specimen	To minimize the risk of cross-infection
Examine the specimen in the sluice using the spoon incorporated in the lid of the sample container	To identify any obvious abnormalities. To prevent contamination
Fill the specimen bottle to at least one-third full	To obtain a usable amount of specimen

Procedure	Rationale
If segments of tapeworm are seen these should be included in the faecal sample and sent to the laboratory	For identification
Dispose of the bedpan and/or contents appropriately	To minimize infection risks
For infants and clients who are incontinent, faeces can be obtained directly from a nappy or pad by scraping it with the scoop of the collecting vessel	To obtain specimen, reduce possible difficulty and reduce potential embarrassment in older clients
Remove gloves and apron and wash hands	To reduce the risk of cross-infection
Ensure the specimen container is clearly labelled and placed in a specimen bag. This should be accompanied by a specimen request form	For correct identification of the specimen

Rectal examination

Occasionally some clients may require a digital rectal examination to determine whether or not they are constipated or whether they have any other rectal or faecal abnormality. Guidelines from the Royal College of Nursing (2000) suggest that only a specialist nurse should undertake this procedure. It is therefore outside the remit of student nurses and other untrained health care professionals. It is recommended that you consult your local policy for further information and guidance.

Monitoring vomitus

Monitoring a client's vomiting pattern along with the amount and consistency of the vomit can help in determining the nature of their condition as well as assisting in helping us determine a client's potential for malnutrition and dehydration, and subsequently their replacement needs. It is therefore essential that this be documented accurately on the client's fluid balance chart (see Figure 5.5) before being disposed of in keeping with the universal precautions (see Chapter 4) and any abnormality reported and documented in the client's care record.

When observing vomit it is important that you note the amount, form, consistency, colour, frequency, whether it is accompanied by nausea or pain, and whether it is related to the ingestion of food or medication. Greenish brown fluid indicates the presence of bile. If the vomit is brown and foul-smelling like faeces, this is indicative of an intestinal obstruction in the large bowel. The presence of blood in the vomit is termed haematemesis and may be bright red, indicating fresh blood from the stomach or upper gastro-intestinal tract, or resemble dark brown 'coffee grounds', suggesting that it has been partially digested.

Projectile vomiting (that is, vomit emitted with force), can occur at any age. Whilst it is not uncommon in children, particularly if they eat too much too quickly, it should be reported along with any other findings as again this may indicate an obstruction or other disorder.

Collection of a specimen of vomit

If a client is vomiting profusely and has not responded to treatment, whilst very rare, you may be asked to collect a specimen for microscopy, culture and sensitivity (M,C&S) or to test for the presence of blood. Testing for blood can be done quite simply by dipping a urinalysis strip in the bowl. Specimens for M,C&S should be collected in a sterile universal container and dispatched to the laboratory immediately, though this test is not considered particularly accurate as stomach contents quite often contain bacteria which may or may not be pathogenic.

What is perhaps more important is that you reassure the client and support them by ensuring that:

- The client is not left alone and has a ready supply of bowls and tissues.
- Their dignity is maintained by providing privacy.
- Filled receptacles are monitored and disposed of promptly.
- The client receives appropriate and adequate anti-emetic medication.
- The client is offered a mouthwash or if necessary assisted in restoring their oral hygiene.
- Any soiled clothing or bed linen is replenished immediately.

In this chapter we have outlined some of the more fundamental aspects of elimination. As you become more senior and more experienced, it is all too easy to forget the importance of these activities to clients in the everyday hub of a busy clinical environment, and, in doing so, delegate them to less qualified and experienced personnel who may not approach them with the same level of awareness, care or compassion as yourself. Therefore it is essential to constantly remind yourself that these are, indeed, crucial daily activities that promote health and well-being, but they require tact and diplomacy, as well as expediency, if clients are to receive a high standard of care.

References and further reading

Brocklehurst J, Dickenson E, Windsor J (1999a) Health Outcome Indicators: Urinary Incontinence: Report of a Working Group to the Department of Health. Oxford: National Centre for Health Outcomes Development.

Brocklehurst J, Dickenson E, Windsor J (1999b) Laxatives and faecal incontinence in long term care. Nursing Standard 13(52): 32-6.

Department of Health (2000) Good Practice in Continence Services. Leeds: Department of Health. http://www.doh.gov.uk/continenceservices.

Department of Health (2001) Essence of Care: Patient Focused Benchmarking for Health Care Practitioners. http://www.doh.gov.uk/essenceofcare.

National Health Service (2001) Effectiveness of Laxatives in Adults. University of York: NHS Centre for Review and Dissemination.

Powell M, Rigby D (2000) Management of bowel dysfunction. Nursing Standard 14(47): 47-51.

Pratt RJ, Pellowe CM, Loveday HP (2001) Epic Phase 1: The Development of National Evidence Based Guidelines for Preventing Hospital Acquired Infections Associated with the Use of Short-term Indwelling Catheters in Acute Care. http://www.epic.tvu.ac.uk.

Royal College of Nursing (2000) Digital Rectal Examination and Manual Removal of Faeces - Guidance for Nurses. London: Royal College of Nursing.

Smeltzer SC, Bare BG (2000) Brunner & Suddarth's Textbook of Medical-Surgical Nursing, 9th edn. Philadelphia, PA: Lippincott.

Tate S, Cook H (1996a) Post-operative nausea and vomiting 1: physiology and aetiology. British Journal of Nursing 5(16): 962-73.

Tate S, Cook H (1996b) Post-operative nausea and vomiting 2: management and treatment. British Journal of Nursing 5(17): 1032-39.

Walsh M (2002) Watson's Clinical Nursing and Related Sciences, 6th edn. London: Ballière Tindall.

Wilson EM, Darby J (2001) Abdominal massage for adults with learning disabilities. Nursing Times Plus 97(30): 61-2.

Wilson M (1996) Control of infection in catheterisation. Nurse Prescriber/Community Nurse March: 31-2.

Winn C (1996) Basing catheter care on research principles. Nursing Standard 10(18): 38-40.

Winney J (1998) Constipation. Nursing Standard 13(11): 49-53, 55-6.

Chapter 9
Maintaining body temperature

Sheila Lees and Penelope Ann Hilton

Introduction

Most of the time adults are unaware of their body temperature because it usually remains at a constant, comfortable level. A special regulating centre in the brain, the hypothalamus, carefully balances the amount of heat produced and the amount lost by the body by, for example, making us sweat or shiver. Control of temperature in this way is part of maintaining homeostasis of the body. Adults are therefore referred to as being 'homeothermic', that is, able to maintain their core body temperature at a constant level regardless of the external temperature (see Figure 9.1). As can be seen their skin temperature can be several degrees higher or lower than the core temperature without affecting overall body function.

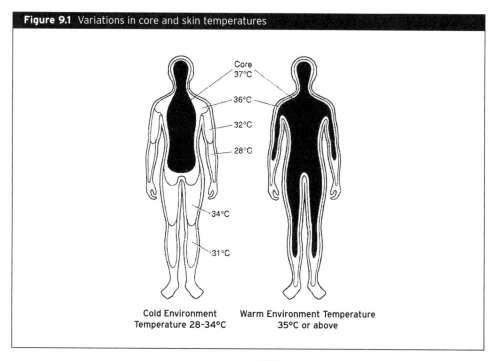

Figure 9.1 Variations in core and skin temperatures

Core
37°C

36°C

32°C

28°C

34°C

31°C

Cold Environment
Temperature 28-34°C

Warm Environment Temperature
35°C or above

In infants and children, however, the control centre is not fully developed. This therefore means that there is a potential for wide variations in body temperature; this is why it is crucial that parents or carers monitor constantly the temperature of infants and children and make adjustments to their clothing and environment on their behalf.

Normal body temperature is subject to variation over the 24-hour day, in keeping with the circadian rhythm (sometimes known as diurnal variation). It starts to rise at about 06.00 hours until 11.00 hours. After 11.00 hours it levels out until about 17.00 hours, by which time it may have risen 0.5–0.7°C from early morning. It then starts to fall again in the early hours of the morning, when body temperature is at its lowest. This is why when we undertake night duty we usually feel quite cold around 03.00 hours and often feel the need to have a warm drink, eat or go for a walk round the ward or department.

The factors that may affect body temperature include:

- *physical*, for example illness, infection, gender, age, metabolic rate
- *psychological* such as emotion, stress and anxiety
- *sociocultural* including exercise, activity, recreational drugs
- *environmental*, for example time of day, severe heat or cold
- *politico-economic*, for instance lack of finances for heating or occupation.

Common terminology

Apyrexia	A normal body temperature
Body temperature	Represents the balance between the heat produced by the body and the heat lost
Circadian rhythm	Sleep cycle (body temperature is lower at different times of the sleep cycle)
Conduction	The transmission of heat from one object to another
Convection	The transmission of heat by movement of the heat through a liquid or gas
Core temperature	The temperature of the deep tissues and organs within the cranial, thoracic and abdominal cavities
Evaporation	To lose heat through moisture, i.e. sweating
Frenulum	The thin membrane anchoring the tongue to the soft palate
Heat stroke	A potentially serious condition produced by prolonged exposure to excessive temperatures, which can lead to coma and death
Homeostasis	Maintenance of a constant but dynamic internal environment

Hyperpyrexia	A very high body temperature
Hypothermia	A very low body temperature
Metabolic rate	The speed at which the body's internal mechanisms are functioning
Pyrexia	A high body temperature
Surface temperature	Temperature of the skin surface (rises and falls in response to the environment)

Normal body temperature

The following levels may vary slightly in different textbooks, but the following is intended to offer a simple, useful guide.

Normal range	=	36-37ºC
Pyrexia	=	38-40ºC
Hyperpyrexia	=	40.1ºC and above
Heat stroke	=	Usually occurs around 41-42ºC
Death	=	43ºC and above
Hypothermia	=	35ºC and below
Death	=	20ºC

The range of normal through to abnormal body temperature is shown in Figure 9.2.

Figure 9.2 Range of body temperatures

°C	Celsius measurement
43	Client does not usually survive
42 41	**Hyperpyrexia**
40 39 38	**Pyrexia**
37 36	Range of normal temperatures
35 34 33 32 31 30 29 28	**Hypothermia**
27 26 25	Client does not usually survive

The sites that can be used to monitor temperature are:

- the axilla (axillary)
- the mouth (orally)
- the tympanic membrane (inner ear, aural)
- the rectum (rectally)
- the skin.

Great care should be taken when selecting the site. Whilst the rectal route is considered the most accurate because of its proximity to the core of the body it is obviously the least convenient, the most invasive and carries a number of risks not least the potential to perforate the rectum. It is therefore the least-used site but the best option when a very accurate measurement is required, for example in cases of hypothermia.

For many years the mouth has been the most commonly used site in adults, but care must be taken to ensure that the thermometer is placed firmly in the pocket to the side of the frenulum below the tongue and that the client is fully orientated and co-operative; confused or disorientated clients may bite or try to swallow it. This site is therefore not recommended in children unless they are fully compliant, nor should it be used for measuring the temperature of breathless patients or patients who suffer from epilepsy. When using this site it is also important to check that the client has not just had a hot or cold drink as this can significantly affect the measurement.

The axilla and groin are useful and less dangerous but are less efficient, particularly in clients who are obese or very thin, as good skin contact is essential for accurate measurement.

The tympanic membrane has become by far the most common site for taking temperatures, as it is easily accessible, least invasive and most speedy. Accuracy does, however, rely on the operator fully occluding the aural canal.

Whichever route is selected, continuity is important, as the measurement can vary by between 0.5 and 4.0°C depending on the site used.

Methods of temperature measurement

Clinical mercury thermometers

Traditional mercury thermometers have been used for many years in clinical settings and may be used in the mouth, the axilla or the rectum. Although they are familiar to nurses and clients, their use has declined in recent years due to the potential hazards of mercury spillage and broken glass. There is also controversy surrounding accuracy of measurement and the length of time a mercury thermometer needs to be left in place. Types available include oral, rectal and subnormal (those that record below 35°C), and disposable covers are readily available to reduce the risk of cross-infection.

Electronic thermometers

These have become more popular in recent years and are often purchased for use in the home. An internal probe is connected to a power supply that has a display unit and bleeps when the maximum temperature is reached. They can be used in the mouth, the axilla or the rectum and should be covered with a clean disposable probe cover for each patient. They take significantly less time to register an accurate temperature than traditional thermometers and have therefore become increasingly popular. Though incurring a more significant cost they are considered a much safer product.

Tympanic thermometers

These are placed in the ear canal and heat is detected as infra-red energy from the tympanic membrane. It is a rapid way of measuring temperature, only taking a few seconds, but there is some controversy over the accuracy of measurement. They are probably the most widely used devices used in hospitals today.

Chemical disposable thermometers

These may be used in the mouth or the axilla. They are usually plastic strips which are impregnated with thermo-sensitive chemicals that change colour with increasing temperature. As these are disposable there is no risk of cross-infection.

Disposable strips

These are widely available from retail pharmacies and consist of individually wrapped strips for single use only. The strip is applied to the forehead until a reading can be visualized on the strip. Whilst they can give a broad indication of whether the individual is hot or cold they are the least accurate and only really serve as a very basic guide as to whether more professional attention is needed.

Assessing an individual's ability to maintain body temperature

The reader is reminded that the assessment of body temperature is part of a holistic nursing assessment and should not be undertaken in isolation without reference to or consideration of the client's other activities of living.

Specific points to consider when assessing an individual's body temperature include:

- *Physical*
  Actual physiological measurement (°C)
  Assessment of possible routes (oral, rectal, axillary, tympanic, surface) excluding those that are injured, uncomfortable, infected or inappropriate
  Metabolic rate
  Shivering
  Body excretions (air, urine, faeces)
  Hormonal influences (women have a slightly higher temperature than men at particular times in the menstrual cycle)
  Circadian rhythm
  Gender (see hormonal influences above)
  Age, infants and older people are more susceptible to temperature changes in the environment
  Has the client recently had a hot or cold drink?
  Is the client obese or very thin?
  Have they recently been smoking?

- *Psychological*
  Emotion
  Stress
  Anxiety
  Behaviour including ability to put on/take off clothing appropriately, and degree of compliance
  Confusion (mercury thermometers should not be used for clients who are confused as they may try to bite or swallow the thermometer)

- *Sociocultural*
  Climate
  Exercise
  Housing/shelter
  Smoking
  Drugs
  Environmental
  Room temperature
  Severe heat

Severe cold
Exposure
Food and drink
Time of day

- *Politico-economic*
  Occupation
  Poor housing, heating
  Poor diet
  Lack of finances for adequate heating

- *Past history*
  Past medical history
  Recent exposure to infection/illness
  Recent holiday abroad

Monitoring temperature

Monitoring a client's body temperature is essential to establish current health status, identify actual or potential problems, facilitate medical and nursing intervention, and monitor client progress.

Equipment

Appropriate thermometer (digital, tympanic, rectal, or mercury) paying due regard to the age of the client, their level of ability to co-operate, local clinical guidelines and contemporary evidence
Designated chart for recording
Protective covers/probe covers
Equipment for disposal, cleansing and disinfection

Axillary measurement

Procedure	Rationale
Wash hands using effective techniques	To prevent cross-infection
Collect appropriate equipment	Remember that only electronic or mercury thermometers are suitable for axillary measurement

Procedure	Rationale
Hold mercury thermometer at eye level, rotating slightly to ensure mercury line is visible. Check mercury is low enough to record the temperature. If not, shake it down in a downward direction, taking care not to hit any nearby objects	For accuracy of measurement To prevent breakage
Explain procedure and ensure client has understood	Promotes client co-operation and informed consent
Screen the bed or close door. Assist client to comfortable position and move clothing away from shoulder	Promotes comfort, maintains client's privacy, prevents embarrassment, exposes axillary area
Place the thermometer in the centre of the client's axilla	To ensure good contact with the skin when the arm is lowered
Rest the client's arm across the chest, advising them to remain as still as possible	To avoid thermometer moving out of position
Leave in position until electronic thermometer signals, or 7-8 minutes for mercury thermometers	To ensure accuracy of measurement
Remove thermometer, read and record result, noting any significant changes	To ensure continuity of care and meet legislative requirements
Remove disposable cover and clean thermometer, adhering to local policy	To prevent cross-infection
Report any abnormal findings	To ensure client receives appropriate care

Oral measurement

Procedure	Rationale
Assist client into a comfortable position, explain procedure, and gain consent	For information-giving and client comfort
Hold mercury thermometer at eye level, rotating slightly to ensure mercury line is visible. Check mercury is low enough to record the tempera-ture. If not, shake it down in a downward direc-tion, taking care not to hit any nearby objects	For accuracy of measurement. To prevent breakage
Cover thermomenter with a disposable cover	To reduce infection risk
Place thermometer under the client's tongue beside the frenulum	To ensure correct reading

Procedure	Rationale
Advise client not to talk, to keep lips closed to form a seal and, if fully co-operative, ask them to hold the thermometer in situ. Leave in place for a minimum of seven minutes	To keep thermometer in place. If the client is unable to hold the thermometer in situ consider using another route. To allow adequate time for the thermometer to register
Remove thermometer, remove cover, read at eye level, record results and report any significant change	To ensure continuity of care and prompt attention if necessary
Clean thermometer according to local policy	To minimize cross-infection

Using a digital thermometer

Follow the procedure outlined above but wait for the signal that signifies that the highest temperature has been reached.

Tympanic measurement

Equipment

> Electronic tympanic thermometer (check for patency)
> Speculum covers (disposable – one for each client)
> Appropriate chart for recording

Identify factors that may affect the reading, for example the presence of cerumen (ear wax), recent facial/aural surgery (potential for injury and should therefore be avoided), hearing aid, or ear infection (the area will be very sensitive and therefore should be avoided; the risk of cross-infection would also be significant were this site to be used).

Procedure	Rationale
Assist client into comfortable position, with head turned towards one side, making sure client has not recently been laid on that side	Client comfort; ear canal easily viewed. If client has been laid on that side, reading may be higher
Remove tympanic thermometer from charging base. Place disposable speculum cover over the probe until it locks in place	For safety; prevents cross-infection between clients

Procedure	Rationale
Gently pull ear pinna backwards, upwards and outwards. Insert speculum into ear canal snugly to make a seal, pointing towards the nose	Straightens the external auditory canal; allows maximum exposure of the tympanic membrane
Depress the scan button on the handheld unit. Leave thermometer in place until a signal (usually a bleep) is heard and the temperature reading can be seen on the digital display	Causes infra-red energy to be detected from the tympanic membrane
Remove speculum carefully from ear. Discard speculum cover into appropriate disposal bag/receptacle by pressing ejection button	Client comfort; safety; prevents cross-infection
Return handheld unit to charging base	Automatically causes digital reading to disappear and prevents damage to sensor. Some units also have a built-in security device in that the unit will cease to function after a given amount of time if not replaced on the base station
Record result noting any significant change and report accordingly	To ensure continuity of care and prompt attention if necessary

NB Some manufacturers recommend moving the speculum in a rocking or figure-of-eight motion to detect maximum tympanic membrane heat radiation. *However, this must be undertaken with great care and is not a recommended course of action for the novice. If in doubt seek guidance.*

Rectal measurement

Equipment

> Gloves
> Disposable bag
> Lubricant
> Appropriate chart
> Appropriate thermometer (that is, low-reading thermometer if client suspected of being hypothermic)
> Modesty sheet/towel to protect client's dignity

Procedure	Rationale
Screen the bed/close door	Promotes comfort and dignity; minimizes embarrassment
Assist client into lateral position with upper leg flexed; keep majority of client covered; expose anal area only	For patient comfort and dignity
Apply lubricant to a tissue and dip end of thermometer into lubricant	Minimizes trauma to rectal mucosa during insertion. Using tissue avoids contamination of tube/container
Ask client to relax and take deep breaths With non-dominant hand separate client's buttocks to expose anus	Relaxes anal sphincter for ease of insertion
Insert the thermometer no more than 5 cm into the rectum and hold the thermometer in place. Allow the thermometer time to register (minimum two minutes). Note the reading	To prevent trauma To allow adequate time for the thermometer to register
Wipe client's anal area with a soft tissue; remove gloves and dispose in clinical waste bag	To promote comfort and prevent cross-infection
Assist the client into a comfortable position and record on measurement chart	To promote client comfort and adhere to legislation surrounding record keeping
Report any significant change or abnormality	To ensure prompt attention
Clean thermometer, adhering to local policy	To minimize the risk of cross-infection

Recording and documenting body temperature

Care should be taken to ensure that temperature measurement is recorded accurately to provide a clear picture of the client's condition over time. If done correctly it enables us to see at a glance any change in the client's condition and helps us determine whether or not interventions are being effective, as can be seen in Figure 9.3. If you use an alternative route to the one commonly used in the environment of care it is important that this is recorded on the chart as this may account for any apparent variation, as can be seen on 12/11/02 at 10.00 hrs.

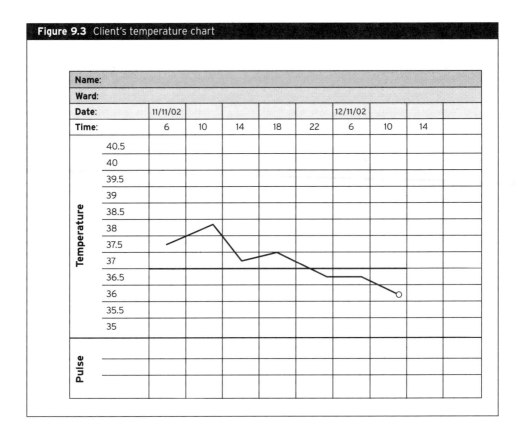

Figure 9.3 Client's temperature chart

Name:									
Ward:									
Date:	11/11/02					12/11/02			
Time:	6	10	14	18	22	6	10	14	

Strategies to raise and lower body temperature

Raising body temperature	Lowering body temperature
Add extra layers of thin clothing or bedding. Multiple layers of thin clothing are more effective than one or two thick layers, as they trap the warm air. Some man-made fibres can encourage sweating and thus may decrease temperature. Cotton is therefore preferable	Remove layers of clothing/bedding. Do not remove all at once or you may cause the client to shiver, which will have the overall effect of increasing rather than decreasing body temperature
Encourage the client to wear a hat or cover the head, as most heat is lost through the scalp	Encourage the client to wear natural cotton fibres as these absorb heat
If possible close any open windows and doors	Use a fan positioned on the client's back as this forms a larger surface area

Raising body temperature	Lowering body temperature
Give the client warm drinks if allowed	Give the client cold drinks if allowed or ice to suck
If possible increase the room temperature	If possible reduce the room temperature or place the client near an open window but not in a draught
Adults and older children can be helped or encouraged to wash their hands and face in warm water provided that they have full sensation. Otherwise there is a risk of burn injury. For this reason hot-water bottles and high-temperature heat pads are not recommended and are indeed banned in most institutions	Adults and older children can be helped or encouraged to wash their hands and face in tepid water. Tepid sponging of the whole body where the client is allowed to dry by the process of evaporation is not generally recommended as this can reduce the temperature too rapidly (see below)
Monitor the client's temperature when actively intervening and ensure that it does not rise more rapidly than 1°C per hour as this can lead to shock. If the client requires their temperature restoring more quickly, this should be undertaken in a critical-care area where the client can be closely monitored	Monitor the client's temperature when actively intervening and ensure in the case of adults that it does not fall more rapidly than 1°C per hour as this can lead to shock. In the case of infants high temperatures can cause febrile convulsions; it is therefore appropriate to reduce their temperature more rapidly. This can be achieved by immersing them fully in a cool water bath
If the client is seriously hypothermic (i.e. a temperature of 32.5°C or below) and continuously monitored a foil blanket may be used with caution, but again care should be taken to ensure that the body temperature does not increase too rapidly. Warmed intravenous fluids may also sometimes be prescribed for this client group but again great care is needed	An antipyretic such as paracetamol may be prescribed if other methods of temperature reduction have failed, though this should not be the action of first resort as it can interfere with the body's natural defence mechanisms

References and further reading

Alexander M, Fawcett JN, Runciman PJ (1999) Nursing Practice in Hospital and Home: The Adult. Edinburgh: Churchill Livingstone.

Baillie L (ed) (2001) Developing Practical Nursing Skills. London: Arnold.

Board M (1995) Comparison of disposable and glass mercury thermometers. Nursing Times 91(33): 36-7.

Buswell C (1997) Comparing mercury and disposable thermometers. Professional Nurse 12(5): 359-62.

Carroll M (2000) An evaluation of temperature measurement. Nursing Standard 14(44): 39–43.

Cutler J (1994) Recording a patient's temperature: are we getting it right? Professional Nurse 9(9): 608–16.

Edwards S (1997) Measuring temperature. Professional Nurse 3(2): 5–7.

Erickson R, DiBenedetto L (1998) Accuracy of Core Temperature Measurement with the IVAC Core Check Tympanic Thermometer, http://www.alarismed.com/library/wp826.htm.

Evans D, Hodgkinson B, Berry J (1999) Vital Signs. A Systematic Review, No. 4. Adelaide: The Joanna Briggs Institute for Evidence Based Nursing and Midwifery, Royal Adelaide Hospital.

Flo G, Brown M (1995) Comparing three methods of temperature taking. Nursing Research 44(2): 120–22.

Fulbrook P (1993) Core temperature measurement in adults: a literature review. Journal of Advanced Nursing 18(9): 1451–60.

Giuffre M, Heidrenreich T, Carney-Gersten P, et al. (1990) The relationship between axillary and core body temperature measurements. Applied Nursing Research 3(2): 52–5.

Holtzclaw BJ (1993) Monitoring body temperature. AACN Clinical Issues in Critical Care Nursing 4(1): 44–55.

HSE (1997) Mercury Thermometers. Health and Safety Executive Occupational Exposure Limits Guidance Notes EH 40/97. London: Health and Safety Executive.

Jamieson EM, McCall M, Whyte LA (2002) Clinical Nursing Practices, 4th edn. London: Churchill Livingstone.

Marks C (2001) Reflective practice in thermo-regulatory care. Nursing Standard 15(43): 38–41.

O'Toole S (1997) Alternatives to mercury thermometers. Professional Nurse 12(11): 783–6.

O'Toole S (1998) Temperature measurement devices. Professional Nurse 3: 779–86.

Peattie P, Walker S (1995) Understanding Nursing Care. London: Churchill Livingstone.

Peters S (1997) Ear thermometry: how does it measure up? Advanced Nurse Practitioner 5(7): 37–40, 72.

Rogers M (1992a) Temperature recording in infants and children. Paediatric Nursing 4(3): 23–6.

Rogers M (1992b) A viable alternative to the glass/mercury thermometer. Paediatric Nursing 4(9): 8–11.

Romanovsky AA, Quint PA, Benikova Y, Kiesow LA (1997) A difference of 5°C between ear and rectal temperatures in a febrile patient. American Journal of Emergency Medicine 15(4): 383–5.

Roper N, Logan WW, Tierney A (1998) Essentials of Nursing. London: Churchill Livingstone.

Rutishauser S (1999) Physiology and Anatomy: A Basis for Nursing and Health Care. Edinburgh: Churchill Livingstone.

Severine JE, McKenzie NE (1997) Advances in temperature monitoring: A far cry from shake and take. Nursing 97. http://springnet.com/ce/temp.htm.

Torrance C, Semple MC (1998) Recording temperature. Nursing Times 94(2) & (3) Practical Procedures for Nurses Supplements.

Watson R (1998) Controlling body temperature in adults. Nursing Standard 12(20): 49–55.

Woollons S (1996) Temperature measurement devices. Professional Nurse 11(8): 541–7.

Chapter 10

Expressing sexuality

Penelope Ann Hilton

Introduction

Sexuality embraces much more than sexual intercourse and gender; it is about desire, demeanour, attractiveness, body image, relationships and the way we choose to socialize. It is about the way we dress, walk, talk and generally communicate with the world at large from a very early age.

As we develop it influences our level of self-esteem and in turn is influenced by our self-perception. As the years progress we come to recognize that we can use it to taunt and flaunt as well as procreate. In other words it encompasses our whole being and is an integral part of our lives, yet, despite a plethora of literature on the topic, it is an area often neglected by health care professionals. This is probably because most individuals in our society find it embarrassing to discuss issues surrounding the topic with people they do not know. Indeed it is well documented that some individuals even find it difficult to broach the topic with people they know intimately.

It is, therefore, little wonder that many health care professionals, not least neophyte nurses, tend to omit any reference to this activity of living during assessment of client needs, unless they are admitting the client to an acute-care setting for investigation or treatment of a specific disease or disorder of the reproductive system, or to a clinic specifically designed for clients experiencing sexual dysfunction. This is with the exception, perhaps, of asking males about shaving and women about their hair and make-up, and, if deemed relevant, possibly their menstrual cycle. Consequently, along with the activity of dying, it is probably the least-assessed activity of living.

Failing to address this aspect of care could not only leave clients with unmet needs but may also be viewed as an omission of care following the Code of Professional Conduct (NMC 2002). This chapter therefore offers guidance on three important areas: assessment, the maintenance of privacy and dignity, and assisting individuals to express their sexuality.

Factors that may affect expression of sexuality include:

- *physical*, arising from alteration in structure, function or processes, not just of the genito-urinary and reproductive systems, for example impotence and pregnancy, but equally the motor–nervous system, sensory system and other bodily systems, for example immobility, breathlessness, loss of sensation, incontinence. Some medications can also significantly affect libido
- *psychological* such as fear, anxiety, depression, sexual orientation, body image and other gender-related issues
- *sociocultural*, for example socially determined norms and accepted behaviours, social pressure arising from perceived deviation, culturally determined norms such as mode of dress, modesty
- *environmental*, for example school, home, work, degree of privacy
- *politico-economic* legislation such as laws governing underage sex and homosexuality, and economic including poverty, overcrowding and unemployment. These latter factors have all been linked to increased child abuse and found to affect libido
- *lifespan* – where we are on the lifespan also significantly influences our sexual behaviours, attitudes and values, for example puberty, menopause

Common terminology

Abuse	Maltreatment, unjust or corrupt behaviour
Asexual	Without sex, sexual organs or sexuality
Bisexual	Sexual attraction towards both males and females
Buggery	Anal intercourse, sometimes referred to as sodomy
Deviant	Moving away from what is generally considered normal, for example buggery
Dyspareunia	Pain during sexual intercourse
Gender reassignment	Sex change
Hermaphrodite	Person, animal or plant having both male and female reproductive organs
Heterosexual	Sexual attraction for someone of the opposite sex
Homosexuality	Having a sexual attraction for one of the same gender
HRT	Hormone replacement therapy. Medication prescribed for some menopausal and premenopausal women to relieve unpleasant side effects that may be experienced during this period of life
Impotence	Inability to achieve an erection
Incest	Sexual intercourse between individuals too closely related to marry
Libido	Sexual drive, energy
Procreation	Produce offspring

Puberty	Period of sexual maturation
Respect	Regard with esteem, refrain from offending
Masturbation	Manual stimulation of the genitals to derive sexual pleasure. A common act of personal exploration in puberty
Menopause	The period in a person's life when the production of sex hormones significantly diminishes, leading to a cessation of menstruation in women and possibly reduced libido and/or impotence in men
Multigravida	A woman who has had more than one pregnancy
Nullipara	A woman who has never given birth to a child
Rape	The act of forcing a person to have sexual intercourse against their will
Safe sex	Using some form of physical means of protection, for example condom, whilst having sexual intercourse or using some form of oral contraception in an attempt to prevent pregnancy
Transsexual	Having the physical characteristics of one sex but an overwhelming psychological identification with the other
Transvestite	Man deriving sexual pleasure from dressing in women's clothes

There are a number of legal issues surrounding the expression of sexuality that are beyond the scope of this text. The reader is reminded, however, that if disclosure of an apparent or seemingly illegal act is made during the assessment process then the health care professional must seek immediate guidance from either a more senior member of staff or the healthcare provider's legal department, particularly where a child's welfare is considered to be at risk.

Assessing an individual's ability to express sexuality

Remember that assessment of expression of sexuality is only part of a holistic nursing assessment and should not be undertaken in isolation without reference to or consideration of the client's other activities of living.

Specific points to consider when assessing an individual's sexuality include:

- *Physical*
  Stage of development
  Gender
  Changes in structure, for example pregnancy, puberty, disease
  Changes in function, for example menopause, hormonal disorders
  Changes in processes

Level of ability
General appearance, for example unkempt, clean-shaven
Present medication
Other illnesses or previous surgery
Presence of scar
Stage of menstrual cycle (if appropriate)
Possible vaginal or penile discharge

- *Psychological*
Fear
Worries and anxiety
Depression
Sexual orientation
Body image
Libido
Level of emotional development
Ability to communicate
Feelings about level of contact, for example touch, personal space
Feelings about changes in structure, function and/or processes, for
    example hair loss following chemotherapy, stoma formation, urinary
    incontinence, impotence
Beliefs about and attitude towards sex and related issues, for example HIV
    and Aids, and receiving a blood transfusion or injection
Perceived disabilities/difficulties
Perceived degree of privacy and dignity
Psychological disorders that might impact on sexuality, for example
    anorexia nervosa, bulimia

- *Sociocultural*
Mode of dress
Level of modesty
Socialization process
Beliefs about social norms and acceptable behaviour
Permissiveness
Any specific cultural considerations
Other societal issues such as hepatitis and sexually transmitted diseases
History of abuse, rape or sexual assault

- *Environmental*
Influences at school
Influences at home
Influences at work
Actual degree of privacy
Preferred level of privacy
Opportunities for sexual intimacy

- *Politico-economic*
  Poverty
  Overcrowding
  Unemployment
  Any influencing legal factors, for example underage sex
  Any influencing political factors

- *Past medical history*
  Any history of illness or medication that might influence ability to express
  sexuality

Remember that assessment at the best of times is a very skilled and complex task that should not be left to neophytes without adequate support, supervision and guidance. In relation to assessment of sexuality, as previously highlighted, this is made even more difficult by the nature of the topic. If you do not feel confident or competent to undertake the task, then acknowledge your limitations and inform your supervisor or mentor of your concerns and perceived development needs, and capitalize on opportunities to observe skilled and experienced health care professionals assessing this area of holistic care need.

Maintaining privacy and dignity

Maintaining privacy and dignity is an integral part of expressing sexuality and is often taken for granted. Think about where you choose to dress and undress, clean your teeth, eat your meals or urinate. Think of the times that you have been glad to get home, close the door, shut out the world and be alone. The times someone has paid you a compliment, or conversely when you may have been rebuffed or ridiculed. Who do you choose to share the more intimate aspects of your life with or even your financial position?

Despite being such an essential component of everyday life, in recent years the issue of privacy and dignity in health care has been the subject of a great deal of bad press to such an extent that the Department of Health (2000) demanded that it be made a priority. Since then it has been highlighted as one of the eight fundamental aspects of care by the Department of Health in its document *Essence of Care* (2001).

Dignity is generally interpreted as meaning maintaining one's position or standing; it is about being worthy of and treated with respect. Privacy, on the other hand, is defined as the right to be undisturbed and free from intrusion. In short it is about confidentiality, seclusion and being away from public view.

Shotten and Seedhouse (2002) suggest that dignity involves:

> being in a position where one is capable: that is, we feel dignified when we have the physical and psychosocial wherewithal to respond appropriately when our capabilities are threatened (p. 247).

Clients tend to feel dignified when they are able to function independently, are actively involved in decisions about their care, and feel respected. Loss of independence or becoming dependent is often viewed as bringing with it a loss of dignity and is what many clients, particularly older people or the increasingly infirm, fear.

Privacy and dignity are interrelated concepts. In situations where clients feel exposed, for example when the nurse fails to ensure that the client is covered before reopening the curtains following a procedure, or when the doctor fails to ensure that the curtains are fully closed before proceeding to examine a client, clients have all too frequently related how they felt disempowered by their loss of privacy. They maintain that this also made them feel undignified, degraded, embarrassed and depressed.

When clients come into our care we often take a great deal for granted. We often expect them to succumb to being dressed and undressed by complete strangers; to bare their all whilst being examined; to bathe, shower, or use the toilet in front of others, without a word of complaint. We expect them to share intimate details about their lives, often to individuals half their age. If we are to expect clients to comply with our many requests then equally we must earn their trust – not just expect them to relinquish their rights because they are ill or in need of health care. It is therefore essential before embarking on a task to ensure that the client is comfortable with your performing the task, not just in general terms of ability and desire but also in terms of specifics such as gender. For example a male client may not wish a female member of staff to see them naked or to take them to the toilet. Equally a female client may not wish to be washed and dressed by a male. If the client expresses such then this should be respected as far as is reasonably possible.

Lack of privacy and respect in the health care arena has become a source of great concern in recent years and has culminated in the Department of Health's stipulating that care delivery must be focused on respect for the individual, in the document *Essence of Care* (Department of Health 2001). In this document they outline seven factors and benchmarks of best practice in relation to privacy and dignity; these are given in Table 10.1.

Table 10.1 Benchmarks for best practice

Factor	Benchmark
1 Attitudes and behaviour	Patients/clients feel that they matter all of the time
2 Personal world/personal identity	Patients/clients experience care in an environment that actively encompasses individual values, beliefs and personal relationships
3 Personal boundaries/space	Patients'/clients' personal space is actively promoted by all staff
4 Communicating with patients/clients	Communication between patients/clients takes place in a manner that respects their individuality
5 Privacy of patient - confidentiality of client information	Patient/client information is shared to enable care, with their consent
6 Privacy, dignity and modesty	Patients'/clients' care actively promotes their privacy and dignity, and protects their modesty
7 Availability of an area for complete privacy	Patients/clients/carers can access an area that safely provides privacy

The following section is designed to raise your awareness of behaviours that can promote or compromise clients' privacy and dignity and thus help you achieve the benchmarks of best practice when caring for clients and their significant others.

Behaviours that promote privacy and dignity	Behaviours that can compromise privacy and dignity
Client-focused care	Organizationally determined care
Determining client preferences	Not establishing or ignoring client preferences
Expanding client's range of abilities	Adopting a paternalistic stance
Promoting independence whenever possible	Creating and/or promoting dependence
Promoting autonomy and involving clients in decision making	Assuming that behaviours acceptable to oneself are acceptable to clients
Being respectful, polite and courteous	Being disrespectful and abrupt
Exhibiting an air of calm unhurriedness	Creating a perpetual air of business

Behaviours that promote privacy and dignity	Behaviours that can compromise privacy and dignity
Listening to clients and their families/loved ones and ensuring accurate understanding (see Chapter 6)	Not listening to clients and their loved ones or misinterpreting what they say
Showing an interest in clients as individuals	Treating clients as sets of symptoms, diagnoses or illnesses
Acknowledging client's existence when attending to care needs	Talking over the client when attending to care needs or discussing treatment options
Paying attention to the 'little things' such as providing a saucer with a cup of tea, providing a napkin with meals, replenishing the water jug without having to be asked, not providing washing facilities following toileting	Neglecting or forgetting the 'little things' or deeming them unimportant
Providing an environment away from the earshot of others when discussing care needs with or about clients, thus maintaining confidentiality	Assuming curtains are soundproof and talking about clients in public areas such as in lifts, corridors, cafeteria, or on public transport
Single-sex care environments	Mixed-sex bays/wards
Ensuring that the environment of care remains clean and aesthetically pleasing	Not paying due regard to the cleanliness or aesthetics of the environment of care, for example failing to clean up spillages promptly or address unpleasant odours
Clean equipment and utensils	Reusing equipment intended for single use. Giving clients cutlery that has residual staining from previous use
Adequate staffing and appropriate skill mix	Poor staffing levels and overreliance on agency and bank staff

Assisting individuals to express sexuality

As previously established, assisting individuals to express their sexuality is essential for the preservation of health and the promotion of well-being, including assisting them to maximize their abilities within the parameters of their perceived physical and/or psychological constraints. There is increasing evidence which suggests that how a child is encouraged and permitted to express their sexuality as a child influences their future sexual behaviour and subsequent expressions of sexuality. For example, exploring genitalia is quite normal for young children; if they are not permitted to do this and are given the impression that it is 'dirty' it may impact on their behaviour as an adult.

In assisting clients to express their sexuality the type and level of assistance will obviously be dependent on the individual's expressed needs and preferences following a comprehensive assessment, and may well include support, education, or referral to more specialist services.

Other factors that might impact on the type of assistance prescribed, as with any other activity of living, will include the knowledge and skills of the assessor, those of the care giver, and the resources and facilities available. Given the particularly sensitive nature of this activity for all concerned, the individual client's wishes must be balanced against the needs, values and beliefs of others without contravening individual rights. For example, a male client admitted to an acute-care setting for a gender reassignment might ask to be situated in a female bay or ward. Whilst it can be argued that we now live in a much more liberated society than our forefathers, this clearly has the potential to compromise other clients and therefore it may be impossible to grant the request. The most ethically sound solution in this instance would be to offer this client a single room with en-suite facilities.

The ways in which we can assist clients express their sexuality are given below.

Abuse	Clearly the management of abuse is a specialized field of practice, our role being to refer clients to the most appropriate resource. It is important therefore that clients do not swear us to secrecy, as it may be necessary to share information with other members of the health care team to ensure the best possible outcome. You should make this fact known to clients at the outset of any interaction, to avoid being faced with an ethical dilemma
Attitude	• Be approachable • Try not to appear embarrassed or uncomfortable when dealing with issues surrounding sexuality • Adopt a professional approach • If you feel unable to address these issues with the client, seek appropriate help. Explain to them that you do not consider that you are skilled enough to help but that you can refer them to someone who is • Seek opportunities to develop your skills in this area of care delivery • Do not ignore the client's expressed need, as they may never pick up the courage to broach the subject again

Birthmarks, malformations	These can have a profound psychological impact on an individual, and clients may look to the health care professional for reassurance and support. We can assist by always being prepared for the unexpected and not showing abhorrence. Have awareness that clients often watch our faces for non-verbal indicators of disgust or acceptance. If the perceived defect is clearly causing great anxiety for the individual, it is often possible to refer the client for surgery or counselling
Chemotherapy/ radiotherapy	Clients prescribed chemotherapy and/or radiotherapy are often very worried about the actual and potential side effects of the treatment and whether or not it is likely to make their hair fall out, affect their ability to have sexual intercourse or indeed whether it will affect their ability to have children in the future. Obviously these are very real concerns for clients and, if not addressed, can lead to feelings of panic and even clinical depression. We can assist clients by listening to their fears and anxieties, by correcting any misconceptions, and referring them to more specialized help if the foundations of their concerns are real. For example, arrangements can be made for some individuals to store their eggs or sperm if appropriate
Continence (promoting)	Incontinence of urine and/or faeces can impact significantly on a person's ability to express themselves sexually. Clearly if a resolution to the incontinence can be found then this should be a priority and many an incontinence advisor has either directly or inadvertently restored or promoted clients' sexual relationships. One question frequently asked by clients with a long-term indwelling urinary catheter, and one sometimes disregarded by health care professionals if clients do pluck up the courage to ask, is whether they can still have normal sexual relations with their partner. The answer is a resounding 'yes', but care must be taken to ensure that, in males, an appropriate sized catheter has been inserted to allow for penile erection. We also recommend that the client wear a condom over the penis and the catheter to reduce the potential for infection and trauma. In females the catheter can be fitted with a spigot and discretely secured to the groin
Contraception	Provide education and offer guidance regarding the variety of methods available, in keeping with clients' cultural and religious beliefs as appropriate
Cultural and religious needs	Develop a sound understanding of differing cultural and religious beliefs, values and expectations in relation to expressing sexuality. For example, Hindu women prefer to be treated by female staff; Islam requires that followers keep the whole of the body covered; Jewish men do not usually like women to touch them or be in attendance when sick; Roman Catholics do not support termination of pregnancy or in-vitro fertilization, and only support certain methods of contraception
Disfigurement following a burn injury	Assistance is largely the same as below, though it may be useful to know that remedial beauticians can often be of great value to some clients, particularly those with facial injuries, in guiding and teaching them how to apply make-up to improve their overall aesthetic appearance
Disfigurement following surgery (perceived)	For some clients, surgery, such as mastectomy, stoma formation, removal of a testicle or hysterectomy, can have a profound impact on their body image. We can assist clients in adapting to these significant bodily changes by ensuring good preparation prior to surgery: by involving them in the decision processes; by giving them time to come to terms with their situation; by introducing them to other clients who have already undergone and adapted to similar sets of circumstances; and by giving them time to voice their concerns, fears and anxieties. We can also help by putting them in touch with local self-help groups and associations. The relevant clinical nurse specialist is usually an excellent resource for such contacts and can also be invaluable in helping clients to readjust

Dress in appropriate attire	Assist clients to select appropriate attire, paying due regard to individual preferences and contexts of care. Parents often express the sexuality of their child through their choice of clothing, for example dressing their baby boy in blue, and this should be respected
Eliminating	Health professionals often make assumptions that clients can urinate or defecate in the presence of others or with a very thin partition such as a curtain for privacy. They also frequently expect clients to balance precariously on bedpans on occasions. Clearly this is not normal behaviour. Nor is it normal for most adults to require that a stranger wipe their peri-anal area, let alone one of the opposite sex. It is essential, therefore, that we allow clients choice in the how, when, where and with whom of care, without taking offence or foisting ourselves on them merely because we are 'professionals', thus promoting privacy and dignity
Menopause	Similar to puberty, the menopause signals a number of physiological and psychological changes in both males and females that can impact on an individual in varying degrees. Assisting individuals through this natural time may take the form of educating them about the process and the variety of interventions available that might help with some of the common problems experienced, such as hot flushes, osteoporosis and forgetfulness. For others, empathy, a listening ear, and reassurance that the individual is not going mad, but that this is a very normal process, may be all that is required
Menstruation	Ensure adequate provision of sanitary wear and provide the means for discreet disposal. If possible, anticipate needs to reduce embarrassment
Personal hygiene	Assist clients to maintain their personal hygiene (see Chapter 3), paying particular attention to hair, nails, desire to wear make-up, use of perfume or aftershave, etc. in keeping with client preferences
Personal space	Do not invade a client's personal space except with their express permission unless failure to do so would result in client harm
Physical contact	Encourage and, if necessary, facilitate clients' pursuance of normal physical contact with their loved ones and significant others. Almost all close relationships involve handholding, touching, kissing, cuddling and other shows of affection. In some instances this may necessitate the provision of an environment of privacy, depending on the nature of the act, the circumstances and the individuals involved
Puberty	During puberty individuals experience a whole host of emotions, for example anger, resentment and frustration, as well as having to contend with changes in bodily function such as the 'breaking of the voice' in young males or the onset of the menstrual cycle in young women. The most common form of assistance we can offer at this difficult time is education and support, not just for the client but also for family members who may be finding it very difficult to understand some of the behaviour exhibited, particularly if the individual is becoming aggressive or self-harming. Often it can help the young person to talk to a health care professional rather than those closest to them, and doing so can sometimes help to avert aggressive outbursts by providing what they perceive as a more objective outlet for their feelings and frustrations. It is important, however, that we acknowledge our limitations and refer the client to more specialist help as appropriate, particularly if the client is manifesting a clear disorder such as anorexia nervosa or bulimia. It is useful therefore to develop a basic level of knowledge and understanding of such disorders. This can then help us to recognize those clients in need of more specialist help

Reviewing and evaluating care	Ensure that care needs are reviewed and evaluated regularly, particularly if the client's condition or circumstances change or if the prescribed care does not appear to be effective
Self-examination	An area of significant concern to many individuals is the likelihood of developing cancer of the breast or the genitalia. We can empower clients by informing them of the importance of self-examination and teaching them how to undertake this effectively. A variety of education leaflets can generally be accessed at your local Health-Promotion Unit
Sexual intercourse	Whilst this may not appear pertinent or a necessary consideration for the majority of clients in our care it would be inappropriate to make assumptions without adequate assessment. For some clients, particularly those in long-term care facilities, the need to sustain sexual relationships can prove particularly problematic. It is therefore essential that staff address the issue with clients in a diplomatic and caring manner and assist in facilitating the maintenance of such relationships by, for example, providing a private and secure space free from likely disturbances. For other clients, it may simply be a need for information or education, such as the 42-year-old gentleman admitted following a myocardial infarction (heart attack) who is desperately worried that he will not be able to resume a normal sexual relationship with his wife. Some individuals may need more specialized assistance and to this end it is helpful to build up your resources by becoming familiar with the specialists in your locality such as the sex therapist, clinical nurse specialists, clinical psychologists, etc. so that you can make appropriate referrals
Sexual orientation	Be accepting of alternative lifestyles in keeping with the laws of the land and code of professional conduct
Toys	Children often express sexuality in their play, for example guns, cars, prams, dolls and association with male or female role models such as 'Barbie Dolls' or 'Action Man'. Sometimes this notion can be exploited to teach children about issues surrounding sex and sexuality

References and further reading

Albarran J (2000) Time to embrace the concepts of sexuality and sexual health in critical care nursing practice? Nursing in Critical Care 5(5): 213–4.

Arthure W (1999) Altered body image and patient care. Assignment 5(4): 11–18.

Atkinson K (1997) Incorporating sexual health into catheter care. Professional Nurse 13(3): 146–8.

Aylott J (1999) Learning disabilities. Is the sexuality of people with a learning disability being denied? British Journal of Nursing 8(7): 438–42.

Bauer M (1999) Global aging. Their only privacy is between their sheets: privacy and the sexuality of elderly nursing home residents. Journal of Gerontological Nursing 25(8): 37–41.

Billington R, Hockey J, Strawbridge S (1998) Exploring Self and Society. London: Macmillan.

Chur-Hansen A (2002) Preferences for female and male nurses: the role of age, gender and previous experience. Journal of Advanced Nursing 37(2): 192–8.

Clifford D (1998) Psychosexual awareness in everyday nursing. Nursing Standard 12(39): 42–5.

Cort E (1998) Nurses' attitudes to sexuality in caring for cancer patients. Nursing Times 94(42): 54–6.

Deakin G, Kirkpatrick L (1987) Sexual problems and their treatment. Nursing 3(19): 709–14.

Department of Health (1999) Caldicott Guidelines (Health Service Circular HSC 1999/012). London: Department of Health.

Department of Health (2000) The NHS Plan: A plan for investment, a plan for reform. London: Department of Health.

Department of Health (2001) The Essence of Care: Patient-focused Benchmarking for Health Care Professionals. London: Department of Health.

Dimond B (1999) Patients' rights, responsibilities and the nurse, 2nd edn. Salisbury: Quay Books.

Earle S (2001) Disability, facilitated sex and the role of the nurse. Journal of Advanced Nursing 36(3): 433–40.

Evans G (1999) Sexuality in old age: why it must not be ignored by nurses. Nursing Times 95: 46–8.

Gallagher A, Seedhouse D (2002) Dignity in care: the views of patients and relatives. Nursing Times 98(43): 38–40.

Gamlin R (1999) Sexuality: a challenge for nursing practice. Nursing Times 95(7): 48–50.

Greener D, Reagan P (1986) Sexuality: knowledge and attitudes of student nurse-midwives. Journal of Nurse-Midwifery 31(1): 30–7.

Haddock J (1996) Toward further clarification of the concept 'dignity'. Journal of Advanced Nursing 24(5): 924–31.

Health Advisory Service 2000 (1998) Not because they are old. London: Health Advisory Service.

Hilton PA (1995) Nursing as perceived by patients, MMedSci Dissertation, University of Sheffield.

Human Rights Act (1998) London: HMSO. www.hmso.gov.uk/acts1998.

Jakobsson L, Hallberg IR (2000) Experiences of micturition problems, indwelling catheter treatment and sexual life consequences in men with prostate cancer. Journal of Advanced Nursing 31(1): 59–67.

Jamieson S (2001) Communicating on sex, sexuality and sexual health. Primary Health Care 11(5): 14–5.

LeMone P, Jones D (1997) Nursing assessment of altered sexuality: a review of salient factors and objective measures. Nursing Diagnosis 8(3): 120–8.

MacArthur A (1996) Sexuality and stoma. Nursing Times 92(39): 34–5.

MacKereth C (1996) Assessing the sexual health needs of young people. Health Visitor 69(4): 144–6.

Maris ED (1994) Concept clarification in professional practice – dignity. Journal of Advanced Nursing 19(5): 947–53.

McAree J (1987) Child abuse: a family affair. Nursing Times, 22 April: 26–30.

McCann E (2000) The expression of sexuality in people with psychosis: breaking the taboos. Journal of Advanced Nursing 32(1): 132–8.

Meerabeau L (1999) The management of embarrassment and sexuality in health care. Journal of Advanced Nursing 29(6): 1507–13.

Moody HR (1998) Why dignity in old age matters. Journal of Gerontological Social Work 29(2/3): 12–38.

Nichol MJ, Manoharan H, Marfell-Jones MJ, Meha-Hoerera K, Milne R, O'Connell M, Olliver J, Teekman B (2002) Issues in adolescent health: a challenge for nursing. Contemporary Nurse 12(2): 155.

NMC (2002) Code of Professional Conduct. London: Nurses and Midwives Council. Also accessible at http://www.nmc-uk.org.

Nye RA (1999) Sexuality. Oxford: University Press.

Oxford University Press (2002) Oxford English Dictionary. Oxford: Oxford University Press.

Palmer H (1998) Exploring sexuality and sexual health in nursing. Professional Nurse 14(1): 15–17.

Roper N, Logan WW, Tierney A (2000) The Roper-Logan-Tierney Model of Nursing. Edinburgh: Churchill Livingstone.

Shotten L, Seedhouse D (1998) Practical dignity in caring. Nursing Ethics 5(3): 246–55.

Sprunk E, Alteneder RR (2000) The impact of an ostomy on sexuality. Clinical Journal of Oncology Nursing 4(2): 85–90.

Thomas B, Hardy S (eds) (1997) Stuart and Sundeen's Mental Health Nursing – Principles and Practice. London: CV Mosby.

UKCC (1996) Guidelines for Professional Practice. London: UKCC.

van Ooijen E (1995) How illness may affect patients' sexuality. Nursing Times 91(23): 36–7.

van Ooijen E (1996) Learning to approach patients' sexuality as part of holistic care. Nursing Times 92(36): 44–5.

Wheeler PN (2001) Learning disability nursing. Sexuality: meaning and relevance to learning disability nurses. British Journal of Nursing 10(14): 920.

Chapter 11

Working and playing

Samantha Athorn and Penelope Ann Hilton

Introduction

The activities of work and play, and the ability of the individual to undertake these, form a significant part of a person's life and yet are so often neglected by health care professionals in the everyday milieu of caring. What are generally perceived to be the more 'acute' needs, and therefore more 'important', tend to take precedence.

To help develop a greater appreciation of the importance of work and play, consider for a moment an infant at birth. They are able to see, to hear and to perform very simple reflex movements such as grasping an object placed in their hand. However, whether they reach any further predicted development milestones (see Table 11.1) or their individual potential (as for example in a child with profound learning difficulty), is largely dependent on how they are socialized and the degree to which they are encouraged to play.

As a point of note, development charts, such as the one illustrated in Table 11.1, should be viewed with caution, as children sometimes develop some skills at the expense of others, and when under stress can exhibit developmental regression to previous developmental milestones, particularly noticeable during admission to hospital. Remember, play is extremely important to the normal development of a child and if they are denied this activity they will certainly not reach their full potential either physically or mentally. It is also an important activity from the health professional's perspective as it provides a medium through which to develop a therapeutic relationship whilst also creating a child-friendly environment. Information about the child's understanding of what is about to happen to them, such as insertion of an intravenous infusion or perhaps a visit to theatre, can often be obtained as the child plays, when their fears and anxieties come to light.

Once we have developed our dexterity and movement within the given 'norms', along with socially acceptable behaviour, it is expected that we will then go on to become self-sufficient and eventually 'fly the nest'. Being able to work is therefore essential to provide an income to support ourselves, and, of course, any offspring we might choose to procreate.

Table 11.1 Child development chart

Age	Mobility	Uses	Social skills
4 weeks	Sleeps most of the time. Lies with head to the side	Grasps fingers when palm touched	Watches mum's face intently and begins to smile at 5-6weeks
6 months	Can hold head and back straight. Will sit up with support	Uses the whole of the hand to grasp objects placed in palm and can pass things from one hand to the other	Puts everything in mouth and turns to the sound of a familiar voice
9 months	Tries to crawl on all fours and can stand for short period with support	Can grasp, uses thumb and index finger	Can hold bottle or cup. Shouts to attract attention
12 months	Will attempt to walk with one or both hands held	Deliberately drops toys and watches them fall	Holds out arms and feet when dressing. Understands some simple requests
18 months	Can throw a ball and get up and down stairs holding the rail	Can build a tower of three objects and can scribble	Can use a spoon and advise when needing toilet
2 years	Can open doors, run around and kick a ball without falling over	Can build a tower six cubes high and turn the pages of book one at a time	Can put on socks and shoes, make simple sentences and ask for food or drink
3 years	Can walk on tiptoes and ride a tricycle. Uses alternate feet to climb stairs	Can copy lines and circles and make a bridge with objects	Can use a fork. Starts to share things and play with others
4 years	Can hop on one foot and climb ladders	Can copy some letters and draw a person or house	Can dress and undress. Uses grammar in speech. Language fully comprehensible
5 years	Able to skip and dance to music	Can copy squares, triangles and most letters and can write some letters without prompting	Can wash and dry own face, use a knife and can act out stories

How often or how long we choose to work in any given period is predominantly self-determined and usually depends on our preferences, abilities and desired lifestyle, most of us electing to strike a balance between work, rest and play. Indeed there is now an increasing amount of evidence to suggest that a lack of such balance in our lives leads, in the longer term, to ill health and possibly premature death. Play thus remains important, even in adulthood.

Such then is our life until we reach our retirement – the age predetermined by the State when we can draw a modest pension to enable us to purchase the necessities for simple living for the remainder of our days. Unless of course we have been fortunate enough to be in a position to make alternative provision and thus afford a more lavish lifestyle or even retire earlier.

The current retirement age for men is 65 and for women born before 6 April 1950 it is 60. However, since the establishment of the 'Welfare State', as birth rates have continued to fall and people are living much longer, this has meant that there are now diminishing resources to support this level of pension provision. Consequently the retirement age in the UK and indeed most other Westernized societies is currently under review and the latest proposition in the UK is to raise the retirement age for both men and women to 70 (McKay and Smeaton 2003). Maintaining our optimum health and well-being in our earlier years is therefore clearly desirable if we are to optimize an active, happy and fulfilling retirement increasingly later in life.

We must also remember that there is now overwhelming evidence to suggest that keeping active in retirement prolongs longevity. Therefore many individuals following retirement from paid work choose to undertake voluntary work and continue to contribute greatly to our societal fabric. Indeed, in recent years there has become an increasing reliance on this type of service; consider the Women's Royal Voluntary Service (WRVS) for example. Yet others opt to act as unpaid carers for their young grandchildren, enabling their parents to go out to work. It is therefore important when assessing individuals' work and play that you do not make gross assumptions about older people's contribution to society.

The complexities of how work and play impact on fundamental areas of an individual's life, and indeed their quality of life, obviously vary from one person to another. Regardless of these variances it is nonetheless a crucial activity of living for most people that can have far-reaching effects. These effects continue to go unappreciated or misunderstood by others, including some health care professionals.

For many of us the complex relationship of work and play to other areas of our lives is not fully explored until such times that a change in our health or personal circumstances threatens one or the other. But think for a moment how you might feel if you were unable to do some of the activities you enjoy, like going for a walk in the woods or along the beach. How would you cope if you were unable to socialize with your friends or colleagues? What if you lost your ability to generate the level of income to which you have become accustomed, possibly forever? What if you became entirely dependent on those around you to go out somewhere, to listen to music or even to have time alone? How would your family and other significant people in your life cope? What would be the consequences of ill health or incapacity on your other roles and your level of fulfilment?

All in all, work and play and the ability to undertake these activities are fundamental to our degree of fulfilment and quality of life. This ability may be affected by many health-related factors – not just injury and disease, but also continued treatments for these, such as chemotherapy and radiotherapy.

A full assessment of an individual's work and play activities therefore needs to be undertaken to begin to understand the complexities of how the individual's life is, or may be affected in relation to, these activities. In doing so it is essential to allow the person the opportunity to express their thoughts and feelings, to support them, inform them and to engage them in fully exploring how these aspects of life may actually or potentially change, in both the short and the long term. It is also important to raise their awareness of how their health can be positively or adversely affected by their work and leisure activities, especially if we are to provide holistic care and promote health and well-being. Consultation with other members of the multidisciplinary team can often greatly assist us in determining clients' actual and potential abilities and needs. These members may include occupational health nurses, occupational therapists, remedial gymnasts, disablement resettlement officers, physiotherapists, social workers and a whole host of other therapists working in the fields of such as play, drama or music. It is for us to utilize and involve these individuals in consultation with the client to optimize the resources available.

The factors that may affect work and play include:

- *physical*, such as physique, level of fitness, health status, alteration in physical structures, functions or processes
- *psychological* including depression, fear, anxiety, perceptions of own worth and role in society, degree of motivation, temperament, level of independence
- *sociocultural*, for example social isolation, changes to perceived role(s) in life and ability to fulfil these, values and beliefs, taboos, socialization processes, social class, pressures from significant others, friends and relatives, loss of social standing
- *environmental*, such as climate, suitability of attire, or environmental hazards that can affect health and safety
- *politico-economic* including perceived level of financial security, ambitions for self and others, employed/unemployed, retirement/redundancy, fear of loss of benefits, lack of finances for aids, adaptations and employed help.

The remainder of this chapter gives the common terminology associated with the activity of working and playing; points to consider when assessing an individual's ability to work and play; how to assist individuals to select appropriate work activities; and assisting individuals to select appropriate recreational activities. The chapter concludes with references and suggestions for further reading.

Common terminology

Art therapy	The use of art to promote rehabilitation
Benefit	Insurance of social security payment, for example sickness benefit, income support
Disablement resettlement officer	A person whose role is to assist clients in helping them to find suitable alternative employment within their current range of abilities
Diversional or distraction therapy	Work or play activities designed to distract attention – usually away from something undesirable, for example pain
Drama therapy	The use of drama to promote rehabilitation
Economic status	Level of ability to generate income
Leisure	The time that is free from work in which we can do what we choose in an unhurried way
Music therapy	Sometimes used in mental health settings to facilitate relaxation
Occupation	A person's employment or profession
Occupational therapy	The teaching of specific skills, crafts or hobbies that promote rehabilitation
Pension	Regular payment made by a government or employer to people above a specified age, or to widows or those who are disabled
Play	Occupy or amuse oneself in a pleasurable manner
Play therapy	A child-directed method of treatment used in psychiatry to establish communication with a child
Recreation	Process or means of refreshing or entertaining oneself
Redundancy	Termination of employment by employer as services no longer required
Rehabilitation	The restoring of a person's ability to function as efficiently and normally as their condition will allow following injury, illness or accident

Retirement	The period in one's life following disengagement from employment usually as a result of reaching a compulsory age determined by law
Work	Application of physical or mental effort to a purpose that may or may not be for financial gain

Assessing an individual's ability to work and play

The activities of work and play will be unique to that person; a full assessment of these aspects is therefore essential to ensure that the client is not left with unmet needs. Gaining insight into a client's usual work and play activities and ability to participate in these may not seem readily apparent nor indeed appropriate at first encounter, particularly if the client is seriously ill. However, a brief initial assessment should always be undertaken on admission or arrival, to identify any significant actual problems that may be causing the client anxiety or distress and which can easily be resolved, such as telephoning the client's employer, school or friends to advise of their whereabouts, or contacting the police to arrange to secure business premises for example.

In relation to infants and children, during this initial assessment it is clearly important to involve the parent, guardian, family or main carer. The child may have a comforter or special toy that can be used as a means of relaxing them during the initial stressful period of hospitalization.

A more comprehensive assessment can be completed later, once the client's condition is stable and/or the full implications of the change in their health status are known, or in preparation for discharge. Remember, some clients who have been absent from work or school for a significant period of time may be frightened or anxious about returning to work or school, and these issues will also need exploring.

As with other activities of living it will also be necessary to reassess the client's ability to work and play should their condition change. Examples may include: the client who has an extension to their stroke following admission to hospital; the client whose health status has deteriorated as a result of the effects of planned treatments or prescribed medications; or the client who has become confused or disorientated, as previously planned interventions may no longer be appropriate or indeed safe.

For some clients in employment, financial issues may not be a cause for concern at the outset, as some employers provide full pay. However, they very often reduce the level of payment as time passes, for example full pay for one month, half pay for a further month and then no pay, barring sickness benefit. Also clients receiving a state pension or other state benefits often have their payments stopped after the first few weeks in institutional care. Referring clients to a social worker, with their express permission of course, can often be of great help in addressing financial issues, as well as assisting us in obtaining suitable aids for clients to enable work and/or play on discharge.

Remember that assessment of work and play is only part of a holistic nursing assessment and should not be undertaken in isolation without reference to or consideration of the client's other activities of living.

Specific points to consider when assessing an individual's ability to work and play include:

- *Physical*

  Is the client currently employed? If so, in what type of employment?

  Do they go to school? Have they any study to do or exams looming?

  What is the client's normal/current level of ability? In the case of infants and small children, what is their current level of physical development?

  Do they normally undertake any physical exercise? If so, to what degree?

  Has the client's job/leisure activity contributed to their current illness/injury? If so, in what way?

  Is the client's physical condition affecting their ability to work and play? If so, in what way?

  Are there any potential short-term effects of the changes in the client's physical condition/treatments on their ability to work and play?

  Are there any potential long-term effects of the changes in the client's physical condition/proposed treatments on their ability to work and play?

  Can these be eased or resolved?

  Can any adaptations be made to enable the individual to achieve their normal work and play activities and resume their previous role functions?

  Is it likely that they will be able to resume their normal work and play activities? If so, is this likely to be fully or in part, and how can this best be achieved?

  Would the client benefit from referral to other agencies, for example occupational therapist, play therapist, teacher, disablement resettlement officer, social worker?

  Does the client need any advice or information regarding their work and/or play activities, for example need for bed rest, need for active or passive limb exercises?

  Are there any aids that can be offered to assist the client with work and play activities?

- *Psychological*
  How does the client perceive him-/herself and their meaningful role as an individual in society?
  Is their short-/long-term memory intact?
  What is the client's level of intellectual ability? Are they able to grasp complex concepts? In the case of infants and children have they reached their development milestones?
  How do work and play feature in their perception of themselves?
  What worth do they place on the undertaking and achievement of these activities?
  Does the client have any fears and anxieties about their ability to maintain work and play activities or about how actual or potential changes to these aspects of their life might affect them?
  How can the client achieve fulfilment in respect to this aspect of life?
  How can they be helped to achieve this, particularly if their previous work and play activities can no longer be resumed or maintained?
  Does the client have any specific fears or anxieties related to actual or perceived loss of independence?

- *Sociocultural*
  How do work and play activities impact on the client's role(s) in society and life?
  Will they be able to maintain an independent life in society?
  How will changes to their ability to perform these skills impact on social aspects of their life and the lives of others, for example spouse, children, significant others?
  In the case of an infant or child, or individual with learning difficulties, is their inability to play likely to impact on their development? If so, how can this be prevented or minimized?

- *Environmental*
  Is the client wearing any protective clothing related to their employment or leisure activities? If not, should they have been wearing any?
  Will the client be able to resume their normal work and/or leisure activities?
  Is their home or work environment conducive to the activities being undertaken? Are there any health and safety issues to be addressed?

- *Politico-economic*
  Is the person employed, self-employed, unemployed, retired?
  Do they undertake any voluntary work?
  Does the client have any concerns regarding their current or future financial security or longer-term plans?
  If there are any changes in their ability to work and play how will this impact on the politico-economic aspects of their life and the lives of

others, for example spouse, children, siblings or significant others?
Is the client eligible for any incapacity benefits and do they know how to
    go about claiming these? Do they require a certificate of incapacity?
    Do they require any help or advice about these issues?
Will the client's changing circumstances affect others around them?
If so in what way?

Examining all of these elements is fundamental to undertaking a thorough assessment of how the individual's activities of working and playing may impact on the complex areas and relationships within their life. By careful examination and discussion a full picture can be acquired, and appropriate assistance, help or guidance provided. The consequences of this may be that the individual is better prepared and able to accept and manage their life, and adapt to the necessary changes that this may involve. Also, reducing any fears and anxieties related to these activities of living can sometimes promote a speedier recovery.

Assisting individuals to select appropriate work activities

Occupation is known to play an important role in maintaining health. Individuals who remain in active occupation demonstrate fewer disturbing behaviours, require less help with fundamental care, and cause less stress for their carers. On the other hand, lack of employment and personal achievement has been shown to significantly affect quality of life in clients, particularly those with learning difficulties or enduring mental health problems.

For some clients their occupation may be the very reason why they find themselves requiring health care. Examples are the individual recently diagnosed with pneumoconiosis as a result of working in a coal mine, the person with repetitive strain injury from typing all day, or one injured as a result of an altercation with a forklift truck.

When examining and assisting clients to select work activities the following areas should be explored with the client, and their significant others as appropriate, to enable realistic and appropriate choices to be made.

- What is the meaning and perceived worth of work and chosen work activity to the person?
- What work activities was the person undertaking, and are these still realistic and achievable?

- What effects might changes have on the person's abilities or capabilities to perform previous or other work activities in both the short and long term?
- Does the individual want and/or need to continue to work?
- Has their occupation any direct bearing on their current health status?
- What is the physical condition of the individual? Are their wants/needs realistic and achievable options given the individual's short- and long-term capabilities?
- Can adjustments be made to their work environment to enable them to fulfil their desire?
- Can any other adaptations or aids help in the achievement of work-related activities and are these available?
- What knowledge and skills does the person have?
- Do they have any previously untapped skills?
- Will further education and training be required and, if so, is help and support available (practical and/or financial) to access this?
- Are they aware of their employment rights?
- Are there any other financial aspects to be considered?

As well as seeking answers to these questions it is equally important that we give clients the opportunity to express their individual concerns and fears, and demonstrate that we are genuinely listening, not just providing guidance related to a predetermined selection of what we believe to be a range of more appropriate work activities.

By working in partnership with the client, their significant others and the rest of the multidisciplinary team, we can enable them to make and set realistic short- and long-term goals, help them to accept any necessary changes and, hopefully, assist them in achieving a balance between home, work and rest. Targeting advice in this way can also help to empower the client, encourage decision making, promote autonomy and help them to achieve fulfilment in the work-related aspects of their life, thus promoting their future health and well-being.

Assisting individuals to select appropriate recreational activities

There is increasing evidence to support the view that 'all work and no play' not only makes Jack and Jill dull but that it can also seriously diminish his or her life expectancy. Indeed for infants, children and those with learning difficulties, participation in appropriate recreational and play activities may well mean the difference between achieving and not achieving their optimum potential. Developing an action plan of meaningful recreational activities for clients with dementia has also shown to reduce the speed of their mental deterioration, and has proved useful for clients' post-acute phase of major illness in preventing boredom, creating a feeling of worth and restoring psychomotor function. Assisting clients to select appropriate recreational activities is therefore an important aspect of the role of any health care professional.

Assisting can take many forms, from listening, information giving and supporting them in decision making (and therefore helping them to make informed choices), to actively getting involved by providing equipment, participating or even campaigning for better resources in the community.

Recreational activities generally considered appropriate are those that can help clients maintain and enhance their health, their quality of life and their overall well-being whilst enabling them to feel that they are fulfilling their desires and dreams.

When examining and assisting clients to select recreational activities the following areas should be explored with the client, and their significant others if appropriate, to enable realistic and appropriate choices to be made.

- What type of recreational activities does the client normally engage in?
- Do they prefer physically active or more sedentary tasks and are these appropriate, normally? Now?
- Do they prefer to engage in team activities or do they prefer to undertake more solitary tasks?
- Do they like to listen to music? How can this be facilitated without causing stress, anxiety or interference to others?
- How much time do they devote to recreational activities and is this appropriate, for example the child who normally spends hours in their room playing on a computer?
- Do they like or need to be mentally challenged or stimulated?
- Are there any social or institutional barriers that need to be overcome?
- Can play and recreation be usefully employed as a diversion or distraction therapy, for example when undertaking a wound-dressing change on a child or anxious adult?
- Is the client bored? Do they get bored very easily and therefore require a range of short activities?
- Do they undertake any sport in a professional capacity? Is this likely to be affected in the future?
- Do they have any commitments to any amateur sporting teams or events? Might they consider it in the future?

- Does the client have any disability that needs to be taken into consideration, for example loss of hearing or sight, sensory deficit or learning difficulty?
- Are they able to grasp complex concepts or follow rules?
- What is their attention span: are they able to concentrate for long or short periods?
- Are they motivated, depressed, anxious, suicidal? Are there any issues regarding safety? Of the client or of others?
- Is the environment appropriate for the activity(s) selected? Is the current change of environment likely to impinge on their recreational activities? If so in what way?
- Are there any health and safety issues that need to be considered, for example giving a child who is being nursed in isolation a favourite or very expensive toy that will need to be incinerated at the end of their stay? Or giving a very young child a toy which can be swallowed?
- Are there any other actual or potential problems associated with participating in recreational activities?
- Does the client have a mobile phone that they use for recreational and/or social purposes? Can this still be used in their present environment without causing a danger to others, for example cardiac monitors, ventilators or other electrical equipment in the vicinity?
- Are there any actual or potential problems arising from being removed from their normal family/social circle? Can these be avoided or overcome?
- Is the client and their significant others aware of the arrangements for visiting?
- Does the client use any recreational drugs or other substances? Is this likely to endanger their health or that of others? Are they aware of the legal position whilst in an institution?

As well as seeking answers to these questions and any other deemed appropriate, as with working activities it is important that we give clients the opportunity to express their individual concerns and fears, and demonstrate that we are genuinely listening, not just providing guidance related to a predetermined selection of what we believe to be a range of appropriate recreational activities. Table 11.2 offers a possible range of play/recreation activities for clients from birth to end of life.

By working in partnership with the client, their family, their significant others and the rest of the multidisciplinary team, we can enable them to achieve balance between activity and rest, empower them, encourage decision making, promote autonomy and help them to achieve their potential, thus promoting their future health and well-being.

Table 11.2 Range of possible play/recreational activities

0–4 months	Cot mobiles Noisy toys Soft, brightly coloured toys Tactile rhymes such as 'round and round the garden' Toys with flashing lights or mirrors
4 months–1 year	Smooth plastic toys with no sharp edges, suitable for 'mouthing' 'Touchy feely' picture books 'Press a button and it makes a noise' picture books Large push-along toys Activity arch and/or play mat Door bouncer 'Baby walker' with activity tray at the front Anything to do with trendy toys, e.g. 'Teletubbies'
1–2 years	Pull and push toys Picture book with simple stories Basic shape (triangle, square, star) 'post box' Telephone with flashing lights and sound Plastic mirror Large-piece animal-shape jigsaws Large plastic animals (child makes the correct noises) Child-selected film character (e.g. Mickey Mouse) Anything to do with trendy toys, e.g. 'Teletubbies'
2–5 years	Paints, crayons and colouring books 'Playdough' activities 'Duplo' building blocks Repetitive action rhymes such as 'ring a ring of roses' More than 10-piece jigsaw Complex story books with animal and human characters Role-play toys (cooker, work bench) Role-play dressing-up clothes Sit-and-ride, then pedal tricycle
5–12 years	Actively encourage own hobbies where appropriate Problem-solving games 'Take turn' board games Computer games Socializing games with rules to follow (let them make up the rules if they want to) Group play and co-operative play activities
12–18 years	Computer games, model making, jigsaws, magazines, videos/DVDs, music, nail painting/cosmetics, card games, board games, puzzles
Adults	Crosswords, puzzle books, magazines, reading, computer games, jigsaws, embroidery/sewing/decoupage, watching TV, quizzes, bingo, origami and other new creative activities, cooking

References and further reading

Baggaley A (2001) Human Body. London: Dorling Kindersley.

Baum CM (1995) The contribution of occupation to function of persons with Alzheimer's disease. Journal of Occupational Science (Australia) 2(2): 59-67.

Carmichael KD (1994) Play therapy for children with physical disabilities. Journal of Rehabilitation 60(3): 51-3.

Chisholm D, Dolhi C, Schreiber J (2000) Creating occupation-based opportunities in a medical model clinical practice setting. Occupational Therapy Practice CE, 3 January: 1-8.

Couch KJ, Deitz JC, Kanny EM (1998) The role of play in pediatric occupational therapy. American Journal of Occupational Therapy 52(2): 111-17.

Crist PH, Davis CG, Coffin PS (2000) The effects of employment and mental health status on the balance of work, play/leisure, self-care, and rest. Occupational Therapy in Mental Health 15(1): 27-42.

Gallagher SM, Keenan M (2000) Extending high rates of meaningful interaction among the elderly in residential care through participation in a specifically designed activity. Behavioural Interventions 15(2): 113-19.

Husband S, Trigg E (eds) (2000) Practices in Children's Nursing: Guidelines for Hospital & Community. Edinburgh: Churchill Livingstone.

Johnson A (1998) All play and no work? Take a fresh look at activities. Journal of Dementia Care 6(6): 25-7.

Johnson KA, Klaas PJ (1997) Recreation issues and trends in paediatric spinal cord injury. Topics in Spinal Cord Injury Rehabilitation 3(2): 79-84.

Jolly D (2000) A critical evaluation of the contradictions for disabled workers arising from the emergence of the flexible labour market in Britain. Disability & Society 15(5): 795-810.

Kelly S (1999) Research in brief. Quality of life for people with severe and enduring mental illness in the community: the issue of activity. Journal of Psychiatric & Mental Health Nursing 6(1): 71-2.

Law M (2002) Enhancing participation. Physical & Occupational Therapy in Pediatrics 22(1): 1-3.

Law M, Haight M, Milroy B, Williams D, Stewart D, Rosenbaum P (1999) Environmental factors affecting the occupations of children with physical disabilities. Journal of Occupational Science 6(3): 102-10.

Long A (2002) The role of the nurse within the multi-professional rehabilitation team. Journal of Advanced Nursing 37(1): 70-8.

Mackenzie A (2001) Symposium on improving care of the elderly: training to engage residents with dementia in activities. British Journal of Therapy & Rehabilitation 8(11): 406-9.

Mayers CA (2000) Quality of life: priorities for people with enduring mental health problems. British Journal of Occupational Therapy 63(12): 591-7.

McKay S, Smeaton D (2003) Working after State Pension Age: Quantitative Analysis. London: Department for Work and Pensions.

Primeau LA (1998) Orchestration of work and play within families. American Journal of Occupational Therapy 52(3): 188-95.

Rebeiro KL, Cook JV (1999) Opportunity, not prescription: an exploratory study of the experience of occupational engagement. Canadian Journal of Occupational Therapy 66(4): 176-87.

Reade S, Hunter H, McMillan IR (1999) Just playing – is it time wasted? British Journal of Occupational Therapy 62(4): 157-62.

Roper N, Logan WW, Tierney A (1996) The Elements of Nursing. Edinburgh: Churchill Livingstone.

Savins C (2002) Therapeutic work with children in pain: use of play and art therapy in chronic and terminal pain. Paediatric Nursing 14(5): 14-16.

Thomas B, Hardy S (eds) (1997) Stuart and Sundeen's Mental Health Nursing - Principles and Practice, UK version. London: Mosby.

Williamson GM (1998) The central role of restricted normal activities in adjustment to illness and disability: a model of depressed affect. Rehabilitation Psychology 43(4): 327-47.

Yaggie JA, Armstrong WJ (1999) The use of play therapy in the treatment of children with cerebellar dysfunction. Clinical Kinesiology 53(4): 91-5.

Chapter 12

Sleeping

Penelope Ann Hilton

Introduction

Sleep is generally defined as a recurring state of inertia where the sleeper is unresponsive to most stimuli. It differs from unconsciousness in that the individual can be aroused by the introduction of direct stimuli, such as a sudden noise.

Human beings adopt a 24-hour cyclical pattern of sleep and wakefulness known as the circadian rhythm, which usually becomes established, learnt behaviour by the age of 3 months. Sleep is generally considered to have two dimensions: rapid eye movement (REM) sleep, sometimes referred to as paradoxical or dream sleep, and non-REM or orthodox sleep. Both elements are considered to be important for an individual's overall health and well-being.

During sleep the metabolic rate decreases, resulting in a reduction in the heart rate, respirations, body temperature and blood pressure. Rest and sleep are considered essential to conserve energy, prevent fatigue, provide respite for the bodily systems, promote healing and relieve tension.

The degree of rest an individual needs and/or is able to achieve depends largely on their age and the degree of mental and physical stimulation and relaxation to which they are subject. An ability to relax fully usually results in sleep.

Newborn babies generally sleep for about 16 hours a day whilst most adults sleep 6–9 hours per night – approximately one-third of their life – making it a fundamental activity of living.

Drastically or continually altered rest and sleep cycles disrupt homeostasis, leading to tension, irritability, reduced concentration, hallucinations, reversible personality changes, paranoia and exhaustion.

Factors that affect sleep may be inhibitory or enhancing, and be:

- *physical*, arising from alteration in the structure, function or processes of the body systems, for example pain (inhibitory) or warmth (enhancing)
- *psychological*, for example anxiety and stress (inhibitory) or contentment (enhancing)

- *sociocultural*, for example mixed-sex wards/bays (inhibitory) or in one's own home (enhancing)
- *environmental*, for example noise that may be inhibitory, such as a loud bang, or enhancing, as in soothing music
- *politico-economic*, for example financial problems (inhibitory) or financial security (enhancing).

Common terminology

Circadian rhythm	Sleep cycle
Early morning waking	Regularly waking at an early hour and being unable to go back to sleep. A recognized symptom of clinical depression
Hypersomnia	Regularly sleeping more than 8-9 hours per day. Often associated with weakness, fatigue, learning and memory difficulties
Insomnia	The inability to sleep despite the desire and/or need to do so
Jet lag	Disruption of the circadian rhythm due to travelling through different time zones
Sleep automatism	Sleep walking
Sleep diary	A record of periods of sleep, rest, wakefulness and activity
Sleep latency	Taking a long time to get to sleep
Sleep apnoea	Periods of interrupted breathing when asleep
Somnambulism	Sleep walking
Somnolent	Sleepy or drowsy

Assessing an individual's needs in relation to sleep and rest

Remember that assessment of an individual's sleep and rest patterns is only part of a holistic nursing assessment and should not be undertaken in isolation without reference to or consideration of the client's other activities of living.

Specific points to consider when assessing an individual's sleep and rest patterns include:

- *Physical*
  Age of client: the older person tends to sleep less, spend more time in bed and have comparatively less REM sleep

Gender: men have more disturbances in sleep than women
Hunger/thirst/diet
Frequency of micturition
Any pain and/or discomfort?
Presence of cough or other breathing difficulties?
Do they have any itching or cramp?
Influence of body position, for example unable to sleep on back/side
Daytime napping
Degree of daytime activity/exercise
Physical illnesses that may inhibit sleep and rest, for example thyro-
    toxicosis (overactive thyroid gland), sleep apnoea
Quantity and quality of sleep and rest
Sleep diary
Early waking or inability to return to sleep?
What is the client's normal pre-sleep routine?
Do they normally use any particular relaxation techniques?
Have they been using any hypnotics or sedation?
Are they on any other medications that might affect their ability to sleep
    and rest?
Do they have an established sleep pattern?
Does the patient awaken in the night? If so, why and how often?
Are they able to get back off to sleep easily?

- *Psychological*
  Is the client under any stress?
  Anxiety often causes difficulty in getting off to sleep
  If a child, do they have a comforter, for example a teddy bear or blanket?
  Depression can cause early waking
  Do they experience hysteria or irritability?
  Are they confused or disorientated?
  Fear of sleeplessness
  Fear of dying
  Loss of partner
  Changes in time zones
  Bedtime rituals, for example normal time for retiring
  Boredom/excitement
  Dreams/nightmares
  Feelings of security/insecurity/loss of control

- *Sociocultural*
  Health beliefs/values
  Do they normally sleep indoors or outside?
  In a bed or on the floor?
  Do they seem obsessed about the need for sleep?
  Do they sleep alone or with a partner?

Are they able to sleep in the presence of others?
Disturbances by babies or small children?
Do they normally sleep in the day or night?

- *Environmental*
  Temperature – too hot or cold
  Lights – too light or dark
  Type of bed, chair, bedding
  Amount of daytime stimuli
  Monotony
  Noise
  Incompatible institutional schedules of activity/rest
  Where do they normally sleep?

- *Politico-economic*
  Limited finances
  Employed/unemployed
  Type of employment – physical/sedentary
  Shift work
  Poor heating
  Poor diet

- *Past history*
  Any related/unrelated illness, for example clinical depression?
  Recent long-distance travel between different time zones
  Family difficulties
  Client/carer expectations

Monitoring an individual's sleep and rest patterns

Monitoring a client's sleep and rest patterns is undertaken to identify usual and current ability, to identify actual and potential problems and to facilitate the evaluation of medical treatment and nursing interventions.

Equipment

Clock
Care records or appropriate chart for recording, if required

Procedure	Rationale
Ensure adequate understanding of the need to monitor sleep and rest patterns (if appropriate)	To reduce anxiety, promote client co-operation and obtain informed consent
If appropriate introduce the concept of a sleep diary whereby the client self-documents periods of sleep, rest, activity and wakefulness	To encourage active involvement in the care process
Unobtrusively observe the client throughout 24 hours	To increase the potential for accuracy **NB** Whilst care should be taken not to disturb sleeping patients during observation, it is important to ensure that the patient is indeed sleeping and not just lying with their eyes closed or in a state of unconsciousness
Accurately record periods of sleep, rest and levels of activity	To determine whether a balance is being achieved
Compare your perceptions of the client's sleep and rest pattern with the client's	To maintain a partnership approach and increase the potential for accuracy, as misconceptions can occur. Remember, a few minutes awake at night can sometimes seem like hours, particularly if you are cold, lonely, worried or anxious. Also the quality of sleep is as equally important as quantity. If the patient does not feel refreshed or rested then this needs to be addressed
Monitoring the respiratory rate and pattern can often assist in determining whether the client is actually asleep	Breathing is usually slower, deeper and rhythmical during sleep
Record amount and patterns of sleep and rest. Ask the client to keep a diary of their perception of the amount of sleep and rest they believe they are getting, and compare findings	Legal requirement to maintain documentation and safeguard client through good communications
Report any discrepancies or sleep and rest deficit	To facilitate care planning
If a balance between activity and rest is not being achieved, reassess the client and amend the care plan accordingly in consultation with the client and other members of the multidisciplinary team	To ensure optimum care

Assisting individuals to achieve a balance between activity and rest

Sleep and rest are essential human needs. Assisting individuals to achieve a balance between rest and activity is therefore a crucial nursing intervention. The strategies to promote relaxation and facilitate sleep and rest are given below.

Equipment

As appropriate for the selected intervention.

Strategies to promote relaxation and facilitate sleep and rest	Rationale
Promote a feeling of control over the situation the client finds him-/herself in	To maintain and increase client's level of independence
Provide an environment conducive to sleep and rest by:	
• Ensuring privacy and dignity	To increase feelings of worth
• Ensuring lighting is subtle	
• Controlling room temperature	To reduce environmental stimuli
• Ensuring good ventilation	
• Speaking quietly and avoiding unnecessary conversation in the vicinity of resting clients	
• Wearing soft-soled shoes	A quiet environment increases the likelihood of rest and sleep
• Reducing environmental noise such as telephones, alarms, machinery, banging doors and movement of equipment	
• Giving prompt care	Reduces stress and anxiety
• Prioritizing care needs	
• Planning care delivery to coincide with periods of wakefulness	To reduce disturbances
• Making sure the bed/chair is clean, dry and comfortable	Comfort is conducive to sleep and rest
Adhere to client's established pre-sleep rituals/routines	Promotes psychological well-being
Minimize stress and anxieties	Promotes psychological well-being
Administer pain relief as prescribed, and evaluate effectiveness	Promotes comfort

Strategies to promote relaxation and facilitate sleep and rest	Rationale
Encourage client to empty bladder before retiring	To reduce the potential for waking
Reduce fluid intake prior to retiring	To reduce the need to wake to urinate
Encourage the client to avoid caffeine products such as tea, coffee and chocolate. Hot milky drinks can help induce sleep	To reduce internal stimuli
Encourage the client to avoid alcohol	Alcohol is a stimulant
Discourage the client from eating immediately prior to retiring and eating heavy meals late at night	To reduce metabolism and to promote comfort
Discourage inappropriate daytime napping	To reduce the risk of an inverted sleeping pattern
Encourage daily exercise in keeping with client's abilities	To achieve a balance between rest and activity
Provide appropriate daytime mental and physical stimulation	To induce tiredness
Educate the client regarding the need for a balance between activity and rest, and correct any misconceptions	To aid independence
Offer to stay with the client until they fall asleep, or provide an alarm or monitoring system	To reduce fear and anxiety
Provide cutaneous stimulation such as offering a warm bath, cold compress or massage	Aids relaxation
Employ appropriate relaxation techniques as agreed with the client and rest of the multidisciplinary team (see Table 12.1). NB Complementary therapies should be used with caution as many are as yet unproven	To ensure compatibility with client's wishes, condition and other treatments
Administer sedation as prescribed and monitor effect. NB This should be an intervention of last resort as many sedatives, hypnotics and anxiolytics have undesirable side effects and can be addictive	To prevent harm To induce sleep
Monitor client's pattern, quantity and quality of sleep and rest	To aid evaluation and reassessment of care needs

For children night-time sleep patterns are often hard to establish, and times for going to bed are often arranged around family routines. To avoid angering parents it is therefore important to stick to the child's established bedtime, as re-establishing the pattern later may be very troublesome. From the age of about 4 months a child needs less and less sleep during the day, until about the age of 4 years when no daytime sleep is required.

Adhering to daytime sleep patterns is as important as night-time patterns as the child will become irritable and cross if sleep is denied. It may also then be difficult to get the child to sleep later. Signs of a child being ready for sleep include incessant crying, unco-operative behaviour and irritability.

Finally, as a point of note, waking in the night during nightmares or for a drink is quite common in children and can also occur in ill adults, particularly older clients and those suffering from depression, where early morning waking may also be manifest. In these cases reassurance should be given as these clients are often confused and disorientated.

Table 12.1 Techniques used to relax clients

Relaxation technique	Uses
Aromatherapy	Some are particularly useful if the client is anxious or over-stimulated. Others can help reduce pain and discomfort in some individuals and promote a feeling of well-being (see Table 12.2). Care must be taken, however, to ensure that their use is compatible with the client's condition and current orthodox treatment
Behavioural conditioning	This can help clients readjust any maladaptive behaviours/coping mechanisms that might be inhibiting sleep and rest
Deep breathing exercises	Aids ventilation and circulation, and reduces the individual's potential to develop a chest infection, whilst having a calming effect
Physical exercise/sport	Whilst involving varying degrees of physical activity, which should be determined in consultation with other members of the multidisciplinary team, exercise can actually aid sleep and rest by providing an alternative stimulus to the brain and musculature
Herbal medicines	Some herbs such as lavender and camomile are thought to combat stress and thus aid rest and sleep in some individuals. Care must be taken, however, to ensure that their use is compatible with the client's condition and current orthodox treatment
Massage	Can be useful for clients who are stressed or in pain or discomfort
Music therapy	Dependent on the material selected, can be used to stimulate or relax the individual

Table 12.1 Techniques used to relax clients

Relaxation technique	Uses
Reading	Dependent on the material selected, can stimulate or relax the individual
Relaxation tapes	Encourages systematic relaxation and is useful in clients who are stressed or anxious
Visualization techniques	Useful for individuals who find it difficult to 'switch off' mentally
Yoga	Can be used to 'refresh' the body and mind at stressful times

Table 12.2 Essential oils

	Effects								Cautions		
	Refreshing	Stimulating	Toning	Uplifting	Head clearing	Relaxing	Soothing	Comforting	If pregnant seek medical advice	Not to be used when sunbathing or using sunbed	Do not use on sensitive skin
Basil			•				•		•		
Benzoin	•						•				
Bergamot	•			•		•					
Black pepper		•	•				•	•	•		
Camphor							•				
Cedarwood							•				
Camomile						•	•	•			
Clary-sage						•			•		
Cypress	•										
Eucalyptus	•				•						
Frankincense							•	•			
Geranium	•										
Ginger							•				
Grapefruit	•			•						•	
Jasmine						•	•				
Juniper	•		•						•		
Laurel leaf							•				
Lavender						•	•				
Lemon	•	•					•			•	•
Mandarin						•	•			•	•
Marjoram					•	•			•		
Neroli				•		•					
Orange	•					•					
Patchouli						•	•				
Peppermint	•						•		•		
Petitgrain	•					•					
Rose Otto						•	•				
Rosemary	•		•			•			•		
Sandalwood					•	•					
Tea tree	•		•								
Ylang-ylang						•					

References and further reading

Bouton J (1986) Falling asleep. Nursing Times 10 December: 36-7.

Burney-Puckett M (1996) Sundown Syndrome: etiology and management. Journal of Psychosocial Nursing 34(5): 40-43.

Burton E (1992) Something to help you sleep? Nursing Times 88(8): 52-4.

Calverley P, Fordam M (1999) Sleep and rest. In Redfern S, Ross F (eds) Nursing Older People, 3rd edn. Edinburgh: Churchill Livingstone.

Campbell S, Glasper E (eds) (1995) Whaley and Wong's Children's Nursing. London: Mosby.

Carter D (1985) In need of a good night's sleep. Nursing Times 13 November: 24-6.

Closs J (1988a) Patients' sleep-wake rhythms in hospital, Part 1. Nursing Times 84(1): 48-50.

Closs J (1988b) Patients' sleep-wake rhythms in hospital, Part 2. Nursing Times 84(2): 54-5.

Closs J (1990) Influences on patients' sleep on surgical wards. Surgical Nurse 3(2): 15-17.

Dorociak Y (1990) Aspects of sleep. Nursing Times 86(51): 38-40.

Fox MR (1999) The importance of sleep. Nursing Standard 13(24): 44-7.

Getcliffe K (1988a) Sleepless nights. Nursing Standard 6 August: 31-2.

Getcliffe K (1988b) Sleep of the just. Nursing Standard 13 August: 18-19.

Gournay K (1988) Sleeping without drugs. Nursing Times 84(11): 46-9.

Heath K, Heatherley S, Ibrahim J (1996) Are pre-bedtime routines necessary? Health Visitor 69(5): 181-3.

Huband S, Trigg E (eds) (2000) Practices in Children's Nursing: Guidelines for Hospital and Community Nurses. Edinburgh: Churchill Livingstone.

Kearnes S (1989) Insomnia in the elderly. Nursing Times 85(47): 32-3.

Knott LJ (1996) Insomnia: a serious problem in the elderly. Geriatric Medicine April: 21-2.

McIntosh A (1989) Sleep deprivation in critically ill patients. Nursing 3(35): 44-5.

Morgan K (1988) And so, to sleep... Nursing Times 84(12): 40-41, 72.

Moules T, Ramsay J (1998) The Textbook of Children's Nursing. Cheltenham: Stanley Thornes.

North A (1990) The effect of sleep on wound healing. Ostomy Wound Management Mar-Apr: 2756-8.

Price S (1994) Practical Aromatherapy, 3rd edn. London: HarperCollins.

Redeker NS (2000) Sleep in acute care settings. Journal of Nursing Scholarship 32(1): 31-8.

Richards KC (1998) Effect of back massage and relaxation intervention on sleep in critically ill patients. American Journal of Critical Care 7(4): 288-99.

Rodehn-Fox M (1999) The importance of sleep. Nursing Standard 13(24): 44-7.

Roper N, Logan WW, Tierney A (2000) Elements of Nursing, 5th edn. Edinburgh: Churchill Livingstone.

Smyth C (2000) Try this: Pittsburgh Sleep Quality Index (PSQI). Clinical Nurse Specialist 14(3): 139-40.

Topf M (2000) Hospital noise pollution: an environmental stress model to guide research and clinical interventions. Journal of Advanced Nursing 31(3): 520-28.

Torrance C (1990) Sleep and wound healing. Surgical Nurse 3(3): 16-20.

Trevelyan J (1989) Now lay me down to sleep. Nursing Times 85(47): 34-5.

Wilkie K (1990) Golden slumbers. Nursing Times 86(51): 36-8.

Willis J (1989) A good night's sleep. Nursing Times 85(47): 29-31.

Appendix I

Rapid reference aids

Penelope Ann Hilton

Introduction

This appendix offers an array of additional useful information to the novice health care professional in a readily accessible format. It commences with a brief summary of the *Code of Professional Conduct*, developed by the Nursing and Midwifery Council (2002; accessible at http://www.nmc.uk.org) to inform the professions, public and employers of the standard of conduct required and to be expected of a registered practitioner.

This is followed by a guide to commonly used medical and surgical terminology, including common prefixes and suffixes, to enable you to work out many of the medical diagnoses you may come across in your everyday practice. There are also a considerable number of commonly used abbreviations.

The remainder of the appendix gives common prescribing abbreviations (such as tds and bd); temperature, weight, and height conversion charts; ideal body weight and average height ratios for infants and children; child development chart; a guide to calculating body mass; laboratory values to help you determine whether results fall within the normal range; and, finally, a section on calculating infusion (drip) rates and medications.

NMC Code of Professional Conduct

As a registered nurse, midwife or health visitor you are personally accountable for your practice. In caring for patients and clients, you must:

- respect the patient or client as an individual
- obtain consent before you give any treatment or care
- protect confidential information
- co-operate with others in the team
- maintain your professional knowledge and competence
- be trustworthy
- act to identify and minimize risk to patients and clients.

These are shared values of all the United Kingdom health care regulatory bodies.

(NMC (2002) Code of Professional Conduct. London: NMC (also available at http://www.nmc.org.uk))

Guide to interpreting common medical and surgical terminology

Much of the terminology used in the medical/nursing world uses prefixes and suffixes tagged on to parts of the body, and, with a little thought, the meaning can be worked out. For example:

intra (within) + **thoracic** (chest cavity) = intrathoracic (within the chest cavity)

tonsil + **-itis** (inflammation) = tonsillitis (inflammation of the tonsils)

Common prefixes

a/an	without
ante	before
anti	against
dys	difficult
ecto	exterior
endo	interior
hyper	above
hypo	below
inter	between
intra	within
post	after
pre	before
retro	behind

Common suffixes

desis	fusion
ectomy	surgical excision of
itis	inflammation
lysis	freeing of
orrhaphy	repair of
oscopy	exam by view
ostomy	creation of an opening
otomy	cutting into
pexy	fix or suture in place
plasty	reconstructive preparation

Sometimes different words are used when referring to a particular part of the anatomy. For example:

arthro	joint
cardi	heart
chole	gall
cholecyst	gallbladder
col	colon
colpo	vagina
cranio	skull
cysto	urinary bladder

derma	skin
entero	intestines
gastro	stomach
haem	blood
hepato	liver
hystero	uterus
mast	breast
myo	muscle

nephro	kidney	phleb	vein
neuro	nerve	pneumo	lung
oophor	ovary	procto	anus
ophthalm	eye	pyelo	kidney pelvis
orchis	testicle	salping	Fallopian tube
os	opening or bone	spermato	semen
ot	ear	teno	tendon

These are then often combined with common suffixes to refer to specific surgical techniques as follows:

ectomy - removal by surgery

For example:

adenoidectomy	removal of adenoids
oesophagectomy	removal of oesophagus
hemicolectomy	removal of half of colon
lobectomy	removal of lobe of lung
salpingo-oophorectomy	removal of Fallopian and ovary
splenectomy	removal of spleen

otomy - to cut into

For example:

osteotomy	cut into bone
thoracotomy	cut into chest
tracheotomy	cut into trachea

plasty - reconstructive surgery

For example:

arthroplasty	new joint

orrhaphy - repair of

For example:

herniorrhaphy   repair of hernia

ostomy - make an opening or form a connection between

For example:

colostomy   of colon to the exterior

tracheostomy   of trachea to the exterior

oscopy - viewing

For example:

bronchoscopy   to view the lung

cystoscopy   to view the urinary bladder

pexy - to fixate

For example:

hysteropexy   fixation of the uterus

Glossary of medical and surgical terms

A Abduction	Moving away from the median line
Abuse	Maltreatment, unjust or corrupt behaviour
Active listening	Making a concerted effort to hear and understand the message the other person is trying to convey
Adduction	Moving towards the median line
Aerobic	With oxygen
Aggression	An attitude of hostility
Alkaptonuria	A rare hereditary disorder characterized by excessive secretion of homogentistic acid in the urine
Amniotic fluid	A bodily fluid that surrounds the foetus during pregnancy
Amputation	Removal of all or part of a limb or part of an appendage, for example uterine cervix
Anaerobic	Without oxygen
Anastomosis	The surgical joining together of two organs or vessels
Anorexia	Lack of appetite
Anorexia nervosa	A psychiatric disorder characterized by intense fear of becoming overweight, even when emaciated
Anosmia	The loss of sense of smell
Anoxia	No oxygen reaching the brain
Anuria	Absence of or failure to produce urine
Apnoea	Absence of breathing
Apnoeustic breathing	Difficulty on expiration with an audible expiratory wheeze. Caused by spasm of the respiratory passages and partial blockage by increased mucus production
Appetite	The psychological stimulus to eat, which may be connected with and triggered by emotional stimuli
Apyrexia	Normal body temperature
Arrhythmia	Abnormal rhythm (pattern)
Art therapy	The use of art to promote rehabilitation
Arthrodesis	Surgical fusion of a joint
Asepsis	Freedom from disease-causing organisms
Asexual	Without sex, sexual organs or sexuality
Asphyxia	Suffocation. Occurs when the tissues are unable to obtain adequate amounts of oxygen
Assertiveness	Able to assert or stand up for oneself
Assistance	Requires help with tasks but is also able to undertake some parts of the task independently
Attention	Awareness, mental concentration
Aural	Related to hearing

B	Basal metabolic rate	The amount of energy needed by the body for essential processes when at complete rest but awake
	Benefit	Insurance of social security payment, for example sickness benefit, income support
	Biliurine	Presence of bile in the urine
	Biomechanics	Looks at effects of movement and normal patterns of movement
	Biopsy	Removal of tissue for diagnostic purposes
	Biot's respirations	Periods of hyperpnoea occurring in normal respiration. Sometimes seen in clients with meningitis
	Bisexual	Sexual attraction for both males and females
	Body mass index	A figure derived from a person's height and weight, which indicates whether weight is healthy
	Body temperature	Represents the balance between the heat produced by the body and the heat lost
	Bradycardia	Slow pulse rate
	Bradypnoea	Slow but regular breathing. Normal in sleep but may be a sign of opiate use, alcohol indulgence or brain tumour
	Buggery	Anal intercourse. Sometimes referred to as sodomy
	Bulimia nervosa	An eating disorder in which binge eating is followed by depression and guilt, self-induced vomiting and purging
C	Cadaver	Corpse, dead body
	Caesarean section	Delivery of infant via the abdomen
	Cardiopulmonary	Related to the heart and lungs
	Catheter	A slender, hollow tube of varying lengths, bores and shapes that is inserted into a bodily structure; in the case of a urinary catheter, the structure being the bladder
	Cauterization	Destruction or removal of tissue by use of an electric current
	Cerebrospinal fluid	A bodily fluid found in the spinal column and brain
	Cheyne-Stokes respirations	Gradual cycle of increased rate and depth, followed by gradual decrease, with the pattern repeating every 45 seconds to 3 minutes. Also associated with periods of apnoea, particularly in the dying
	Circadian rhythm	Sleep cycle
	Circumduction	Moving through a circle, in combination
	Clarifying	Making clear, ensuring understanding
	Cognition	Ability to understand
	Colloquialism	Word or phrase used in everyday speech but not for formal speech or writing

Communication	Passage of information from one to another
Conduction	The transmission of heat from one object to another
Constipation	Infrequent and often difficult evacuation of faeces or the passage of hard stools less frequently than the client's own normal pattern
Continence	The ability to retain bodily excrement, i.e. urine and faeces, until such time as is appropriate to eliminate them
Convection	The transmission of heat by movement of the heat through a liquid or gas
Core temperature	The temperature of the deep tissues and organs within the cranial, thoracic and abdominal cavities
Coroner	A person appointed by the Home Office who is required by law to investigate deaths due to unnatural, suspicious or unknown causes
Cues	Things that are said or done which serve as a signal for something else to be done
Cyanosis	Blue tinge to skin and body tissues caused by hypoxia
Cystitis	Inflammation of the bladder
Cytotoxic	Chemicals that destroy cells

D

De-escalation	A term commonly used to refer to techniques for diffusing a potentially aggressive or hostile situation
Defecation	The discharge of waste products from the rectum
Dependent	Unable to help, needs full assistance to achieve task
Deviant	Moving away from what is generally considered normal, for example buggery
Diaphoresis	Perspiration, particularly if excessive
Diarrhoea	Loose and sometimes watery frequent evacuation of stools, with or without discomfort
Diastole	The resting phase of the heart muscle during which the chambers of the heart fill with blood
Dilation and curettage	Scraping of the uterus lining
Disability	Any restriction or lack of ability to perform an activity within the socially accepted norms
Disablement resettlement officer	A person whose role is to assist clients in helping them to find suitable alternative employment within their current range of abilities
Diversional therapy	Work or play activities designed to distract attention - usually away from something undesirable, for example pain
Dorsal	Relating to the back
Dorsiflexion	Bending of the foot and toes upwards
Drama therapy	The use of drama to promote rehabilitation

Dyslexia	Impairment of ability to read with comprehension
Dyspareunia	Pain during sexual intercourse
Dyspepsia	Heartburn
Dysphagia	Difficulty with swallowing
Dysphasia	Difficulty with speaking
Dysphonia	Difficulty in pronouncing sounds
Dyspnoea	Difficulty breathing
Dyspraxia	Difficulty in performing co-ordinated movements
Dysuria	Pain when passing urine

E

Eclampsia	A severe form of toxaemia that occurs in pregnancy and which can lead to convulsions, coma and death
Economic status	Level of ability to generate income
Embolus	A small body, usually broken off from a thrombus, that circulates with the blood until the vessel it is travelling in becomes too small for it to go further. It may also be an air bubble or foreign body
Empathy	The ability to identify with another person and understand their point of view
Endogenous	From within
Enucleation	Removal of eyeball
Ergonomics	Looks at effective use of energy in relation to efficient movement
Evaporation	To lose heat through moisture, that is, sweating
Eversion	Turning outwards
Evisceration	Removal of internal organs or removal of contents of eyeball
Exogenous	From an external source
Expiration	The act of breathing out
Expressive dysphasia	Difficulty in expressing oneself with speech
Extension	Straightening
External rotation	Rolling outwards

F

Fistula	An abnormal communication between two organs or body cavities, for example between colon and bladder
Flexion	Bending
Frenulum	The thin layer of tissue attaching the tongue to the soft palate
Frequency	The felt need to pass urine more often than normal

G

Gender reassignment	Sex change
Gingivitis	Inflammation of the gums
Glossitis	Inflammation of the tongue
Glycosuria	Presence of glucose in the urine

H Haematemesis	Blood in the vomit
Haematoma	A swelling filled with blood
Haematuria	Presence of blood in the urine
Haemoptysis	Presence of blood in the sputum
Haemorrhoids	Protruding vein in the rectal area
Halitosis	Bad breath
Handicap	A disadvantage for a given individual resulting from an impairment or disability that prevents fulfilment of a role in the normal manner
Heat stroke	A potentially serious condition produced by prolonged exposure to excessive temperatures; can lead to coma and death
Hemiparesis	Weakness/paralysis on one side of the body
Hemiplegia	Paralysis on one side of the body
Hermaphrodite	Person, animal or plant having both male and female reproductive organs
Heterosexual	Sexual attraction for someone of the opposite sex
Homeostasis	The automated self-regulation to maintain the normal state of the body under a variety of conditions
Homosexuality	Having a sexual attraction for one of the same gender
HRT	Hormone replacement therapy. Medication prescribed for some menopausal and pre-menopausal women to relieve unpleasant side effects that may be experienced during this period of life
Hypercapnia	High partial pressure of carbon dioxide
Hyperglycaemia	High blood sugar levels
Hyperpnoea	Deep breathing with marked use of abdominal muscles. Common in acidotic states
Hyperpyrexia	A very high body temperature
Hypertension	High blood pressure
Hyperthermia	Raised body temperature
Hyperventilation	Increased rate of breathing
Hypoglycaemia	Low blood sugar
Hypotension	Low blood pressure
Hypothermia	Low body temperature, usually below 35°C
Hypoventilation	Irregular, slow, shallow breathing
Hypovolaemic	Low circulatory blood volume
Hypoxaemia	A lack of oxygen in the blood
Hypoxia	Low amount of oxygen reaching the brain
I Impairment	Any loss or abnormality of physical or psychological function
Impotence	Inability to achieve an erection

Incest	Sexual intercourse between individuals too closely related to marry
Incontinence	Inability to resist the urge to urinate or defecate
Independent	Needs no assistance with task
Indole	A product of intestinal putrefaction
Inferences	To imply or suggest without stating directly
Inquest	An investigation held by the Coroner when death is known or suspected to be due to any other cause than natural death
Inspiration	The act of breathing in
Intermittent claudication	When the oxygen demands made by the tissues in the feet become too great for the occluded artery, a cramp-like pain is felt in the calf
Internal rotation	Rolling inwards
Inversion	Turning inwards

K

Kussmaul's respirations	Increased respiratory rate (above 20 rpm), increased depth, panting, laboured breathing. Causes include diabetic ketoacidosis and renal failure

L

Labelling	A form of stereotyping, for example 'the unpopular patient'
Leisure	The time that is free from work in which we can do what we choose in an unhurried way
Libido	Sexual drive, energy

M

Malabsorption	Inadequate or disordered absorption of nutrients from the intestinal canal
Malnutrition	The state of being poorly nourished. May be caused by inadequate food or deficiency of some essential nutrients, or by malabsorption by metabolic defect that prevents the body from utilizing nutrients properly
Masturbation	Manual stimulation of the genitals to derive sexual pleasure. A common act of personal exploration in puberty
Meatus	The external opening of the urethra
Medical Certificate of Death	Sometimes referred to as the Death Certificate, is a legal document required by the Registrar of Births, Deaths and Marriages before they can issue a form permitting disposal of the body
Meleana	Black, tarry stools as a result of digesting blood
Menopause	The period in a person's life when the production of sex hormones significantly diminishes, leading to a cessation of menstruation in women and possibly reduced libido and/or impotence in men

Menstruation	The periodic shedding of blood, secretions and cells from the uterus of a non-pregnant, fertile woman, lasting about 4–5 days. This usually occurs in cycles of approximately 28 days and is influenced by the excretion of oestrogen and progesterone
Metabolic rate	The speed at which the body's internal mechanisms are functioning
Metabolism	The process by which cells in the body are destroyed and renewed by chemical substances in the blood
Micturition	The act of passing urine
Motion	A term sometimes used for a bowel movement
Multigravida	A woman who has had more than one pregnancy
Music therapy	Sometimes used in mental health and other settings to facilitate relaxation
Myoglobin	Muscle protein that transports oxygen

N

Nocturia	Excessive passing of urine in the night
Non-verbal communication	Communicating without the use of words, for example touch, gesture, facial expression
Normotension	Blood pressure within normal limits
Nosocomial infection	Hospital-acquired infection
Nullipara	A woman who has never given birth to a child
Nutrition	The science related to the food requirements of the body

O

Occupation	A person's employment or profession
Occupational therapy	The teaching of specific skills, crafts or hobbies that promote rehabilitation
Oliguria	Low urine output
Oral	Related to mouth/speech
Orthopnoea	The ability to breath easily only when in an upright position

P

Paracentesis	Procedure involving the puncturing of a cavity wall to drain or remove bodily fluid
Paralysis	Impairment or loss of motor function
Paraphrasing	To express the meaning in simple terms, rewording
Pathogenic	Disease causing
Pathologist	A doctor trained in the detection and diagnosis of disease
Pension	Regular payment made by a government or employer to people above a specified age, or to widows or those who are disabled
Perception	Ability to see and understand

Percutaneous Endoscopic Gastrostomy (PEG)	A feeding tube inserted into the stomach through the outer abdominal wall
Perfusion	The flow of oxygenated blood to the tissues
Perineum	The area of skin between the external genitalia and the anus
Periodontitis	Inflammation of the gums, palate and surrounding structures
Peritoneal fluid	A bodily fluid found within the perineum in some disorders
Personality	Our individual character, our distinctive qualities that make us who we are
Phlebitis	Inflammation of a vein
Plantar	Related to the sole of the foot, as in plantar reflex
Plaque	A deposit of food and bacteria on the teeth, which may produce tartar and dental caries
Play	Occupy or amuse oneself in a pleasurable manner
Play therapy	A method of treatment used in psychiatry to establish communication with a child
Position	Posture or placement
Post-mortem	Involves the examination of the brain and other internal organs by a pathologist, usually undertaken when the cause of death is uncertain or suspicious
Procreation	Produce offspring
Prognosis	Course of the disease, including expected outcome
Pronation	Turning the palm of the hand downwards
Prone	Lying face downwards
Proteinuria	Presence of protein in the urine
Puberty	Period of sexual maturation
Pyrexia	A high temperature, usually above 38ºC

Q Quadriplegia	Paralysis of all four limbs

R Rape	The act of forcing a person to have sexual intercourse against their will
Receptive dysphasia	Difficulty in understanding speech
Recreation	Process or means of refreshing or entertaining oneself
Recumbent	Lying down in the dorsal position
Redundancy	Termination of employment by employer, as services no longer required
Reflex	An involuntary action
Rehabilitation	The restoring of a person's ability to function as efficiently and normally as their condition will allow following injury, illness or accident

Respect	Regard with esteem, refrain from offending
Retirement	The period in one's life following disengagement from employment, usually as a result of reaching a compulsory age determined by law
Rose Cottage	A term commonly used for the mortuary when speaking in a public area

S Safe sex — Using some form of physical means of protection, for example condom, whilst having sexual intercourse, or using some form of contraception in an attempt to prevent pregnancy

Self-awareness	Noticing or being aware of yourself, your actions, your abilities and the impact these have or may have on others
Self-image	The way you see yourself or would describe yourself to others
Semi-prone	Lying on one side
Semi-recumbent	Lying down in the dorsal position with a pillow under the head
Sepsis	Presence of micro-organisms causing toxicity in the body
Sinus	A blind-ended channel or tract
Skatole	A strong-smelling nitrogen compound in human faeces
Sphygmomanometer	Device used to measure blood pressure
Steatorrhoea	Pale, bulky, fatty stools
Stent	An expandable meshlike structure placed in an artery to prevent vasoconstriction and thus maintain potency
Stereotyping	Assigning people to categories based on assumptions rather than fact, for example all fat people are lazy
Stoma	An artificial opening established surgically between an organ and the exterior
Stomatitis	Inflammation of the mouth
Stool	Another term sometimes used for a bowel movement
Stridor	A harsh, vibrating, shrill sound produced during respiration. Usually indicates an obstruction
Summarizing	Pulling together the main points
Supervision	Needs verbal encouragement and observing when undertaking a task
Supination	Turning upwards
Supine	Lying on the back facing upwards
Suprapubic	Situated above the pubic bone
Surface temperature	Temperature of the skin surface (rises and falls in response to the environment)
Sympathy	A feeling of pity or tenderness towards one who is suffering

| Synovial fluid | A bodily fluid found in a joint, for example knee |
| Systole | The contraction of the heart muscle |

T

Tachycardia	Fast pulse rate
Tachypnoea	Increased rate of breathing
Tenting	A sign of dehydration where the skin, when gently pinched, is slow to return to its normal state
Therapeutic	Healing, curative, comforting
Tracheostomy	Making of an opening into the trachea (windpipe)
Transsexual	Having the physical characteristics of one sex but an overwhelming psychological identification with the other
Transvestite	Man deriving sexual pleasure from dressing in women's clothes
Turgidity	Degree of swelling
Turgor	Resistance of the skin to deformation when pinched. Related mainly to age but also to the level of hydration

U

Universal precautions	Locally, nationally and internationally acknowledged guidelines aimed at reducing the risk of cross-infection, contamination or injury within health care settings
Urethritis	Inflammation of the urethra
Urgency	A sudden strong desire to pass urine
Urinalysis	Testing of urine for abnormalities
Urinate	To discharge urine from the body

V

Validating	Confirming, checking
Ventilation	The movement of air in and out of the lungs
Verbal communication	The spoken word and how we speak, including tone, pitch and volume
Violence	Unwarranted physical force or strength exerted with the intention of injuring or destroying another individual
Voiding urine	Emptying the bladder

W

| Work | Application of physical or mental effort to a purpose that may or may not be for financial gain |

X

| Xerostomia | Dryness of the mouth |

Common medical and nursing abbreviations

Whilst the use of abbreviations is generally discouraged, unfortunately they are an inevitable part of everyday life in the clinical arena. The following is therefore designed to assist you in interpreting those in common use.

A much more comprehensive list of abbreviations and acronyms can be found at http://www.pharma-lexicon.com.

AAA	Abdominal aortic aneurysm
ABGs	Arterial blood gases
ABR	Abdominal X-ray
ACLS	Advanced cardiac life support
AF	Atrial fibrillation/flutter
AKA	Above-knee amputation
ALS	Advanced life support
AMA	Against medical advice
AP resection	Abdominal–perineal resection
Asps	Aspirations, for example NG Asps (nasogastric aspirations)
AV	Arterio-venous, for example fistula or shunt
AXR	Abdominal X-ray
BID	Brought in dead
BKA	Below-knee amputation
BLS	Basic life support
BMs	Blood sugar levels (the term BMs originates from the company that originally produced the analysis sticks)
B/P	Blood pressure
BT	Blood transfusion
c/o	Complaining of
CABG	Coronary artery bypass graft
Caes(e)	Caesarean section
CAPD	Continuous ambulatory peritoneal dialysis
CBD	Catheter bladder drainage
CCF	Congestive cardiac failure
CCU	Coronary care unit
CD	Controlled drug
CICU	Cardiac intensive care unit
CIU	Clinical investigations unit
CNS	Clinical nurse specialist or central nervous system (dependent on the context)
COAD	Chronic obstructive airways disease
COPD	Chronic obstructive pulmonary disease
CPAP	Continuous positive airways pressure
CNS obs	Central nervous system observations
C & S	Culture and sensitivity

CSF	Cerebrospinal fluid
CSU	Catheter specimen of urine
CT scan	Computerized tomography scan
CVA	Cerebral vascular accident (stroke)
CVS	Cardio-vascular system
CXR	Chest X-ray
D & V	Diarrhoea and vomiting
DIC	Disseminated intravascular coagulation
DKA	Diabetic keto-acidosis
DN	District nurse
DNR	Do not resuscitate
DOA	Dead on arrival
DVT	Deep vein thrombosis
EAU	Emergency admissions unit
ECG	Electrocardiography
EEG	Electroencephalogram
EMD	Electromechanical dissociation
EMU	Early morning urine specimen
ENT	Ear, nose and throat
ERCP	Endoscopic retrograde cholangio-pancreatography
Epi	Epidural/epidurally
ETA	Estimated time of arrival
FBC	Full blood count
FOB	Faeces for occult blood
FOF	Found on floor
GCS	Glasgow Coma Scale/Score
GICU	General intensive care unit
GIT	Gastro-intestinal tract
GU	Genito-urinary
GWO	Gastric washout
Hb	Haemoglobin
HI	Head injury
HO	House officer
HDU	High-dependency unit
IBD	Irritable bowel disease
IBS	Inflammatory bowel disease
ICP	Intra-cranial pressure
ICU	Intensive care unit
IDDM	Insulin-dependent diabetes mellitus
IHD	Ischaemic heart disease
INR	International normalized ratio
IPD	Intermittent peritoneal dialysis
ITU	Intensive treatment unit
i/c	With

IV ABs	Intravenous antibiotics
IVI	Intravenous infusion
IVT	Intravenous therapy
Ix	Investigation
JVP	Jugular venous pressure
KCT	Kaolin coagulation time
KUB	X-rays of the kidneys, ureters and bladder
Lap Choly	Laparoscopic cholecystectomy
LBKA	Left below-knee amputation
LFTs	Liver function tests
LIF	Left iliac fossa
LOC	Loss of consciousness
LP	Lumbar puncture
LRTI	Lower respiratory tract infection
LUQ	Left upper quadrant
M, C & S	Microscopy, culture and sensitivity
MDT	Multidisciplinary team
MI	Myocardial infarction
MRI scan	Magnetic resonance imaging scan
MRSA	Methicillin-resistant *Staphylococcus aureus*
MSU	Mid-stream urine specimen
NAD	No abnormality detected
NBM	Nil by mouth
NFA	No fixed abode
NFR	Not for resuscitation
NGT	Nasogastric tube
NIDD	Non-insulin-dependent diabetic
NIDDM	Non-insulin-dependent diabetes mellitus
# NOF	Fractured neck of femur
NPU	Not passed urine
Obs	Observations, for example temperature, pulse, blood pressure
OPA	Outpatient appointment
OPD	Outpatients' department
OT	Occupational therapist
PACU	Post-anaesthetic care unit
PCA	Patient-controlled analgesia
PE	Pulmonary embolus
PICC	Percutaneously inserted central catheter
PID	Pelvic inflammatory disease
PMH	Past medical history
POP	Plaster of Paris
PPH	Primary pulmonary hypertension
PTC (and stent)	Percutaneous trans-hepatic cholangiography

PUT	Passed urine in toilet
PVD	Peripheral vascular disease
Px	Treatment
RAKA	Right above-knee amputation
RBCs	Red blood cells
Reg	Registrar
RIF	Right iliac fossa
RIHR	Right inguinal hernia repair
RIP	Rest in peace
RMO	Resident medical officer
RSO	Resident surgical officer
RTA	Road traffic accident
RUQ	Right upper quadrant
RVD	Redi vac drain
SHO	Senior house officer
SOB	Shortness of breath
SOBOE	Shortness of breath on exertion
Sr	Sister
SR	Senior registrar
STD	Sexually transmitted disease
SVT	Sinus ventricular tachycardia
SW	Social worker
TED stockings	Anti-embolic stockings
TLC	Tender loving care
TOD	Took own discharge
TOE	Trans-oesophageal echocardiogram
TOP	Termination of pregnancy
TPC	Total patient care
TPN	Total parenteral nutrition
TPR	Temperature, pulse and respirations
TTHs	Tablets to take home
TTOs	Tablets to take out
TURP	Trans-urethral resection of prostate
TURT	Trans-urethral resection of tumour
Tx	Treatment
URTI	Upper respiratory tract infection
USS	Ultrasound scan
UTI	Urinary tract infection
Us & Es	Urea and electrolytes
VF	Ventricular fibrillation
VT	Ventricular tachycardia
VQ scan	Ventilation perfusion scan
VVS	Varicose vein surgery
WCC	White cell count

Common prescribing abbreviations

Term	Latin	English
ad lib	ad libitum	to the desired amount
bd	bis in die	twice a day
bid	bis in die	twice a day
CD		controlled drug
endo		via the endotracheal tube
ID		intradermal
IM		intramuscular
IT		intrathecal
IV		intravenous
IVI		intravenous infusion
mane		in the morning
mist	mistura	mixture
om	omni mane	every morning
on	omni nocte	every night
pr	per rectus	via the rectum
prn	pro re nata	whenever necessary
pv		via the vagina
qds	quarter in die	four times a day
SB		sub-buccal (under the tongue)
SC		subcutaneous
SL		sublingual
stat	statim	at once
tds	ter die sumendum	three times a day
tid	ter in die	three times a day
top		topical
vol		volume

Conversion tables

Temperature

°C means temperature in degrees Celsius (°C x 9/5 + 32 = °F)
°F means temperature in degrees Fahrenheit (°F − 32 x 5/9 = °C)

°C	°F	°C	°F
34.0	93.2	38.6	101.5
34.2	93.6	38.8	101.8
34.4	93.9	39.0	102.2
34.6	94.3	39.2	102.6
34.8	94.6	39.4	102.9
35.0	95.0	39.6	103.3
35.2	95.4	39.8	103.6
35.4	95.7	40.0	104.0
35.6	96.1	40.2	104.4
35.8	96.4	40.4	104.7
36.0	96.8	40.6	105.2
36.2	97.2	40.8	105.4
36.4	97.5	41.0	105.9
36.6	97.9	41.2	106.1
36.8	98.2	41.4	106.5
37.0	98.6	41.6	106.8
37.2	99.0	41.8	107.2
37.4	99.3	42.0	107.6
37.6	99.7	42.2	108.0
37.8	100.0	42.4	108.3
38.0	100.4	42.6	108.7
38.2	100.8	42.8	109.0
38.4	101.1	43.0	109.4

Weight

1 kg = 2.2 lb	1 stone = 6.35 kg	
1 lb = 0.45 kg	1 stone = 6.35 kg	15 stone = 95.25 kg
2 lb = 0.91 kg	2 stone = 12.70 kg	16 stone = 101.60 kg
3 lb = 1.36 kg	3 stone = 19.05 kg	17 stone = 107.95 kg
4 lb = 1.81 kg	4 stone = 25.40 kg	18 stone = 114.30 kg
5 lb = 2.27 kg	5 stone = 31.75 kg	19 stone = 120.65 kg
6 lb = 2.72 kg	6 stone = 38.10 kg	20 stone = 127.00 kg
7 lb = 3.18 kg	7 stone = 44.45 kg	21 stone = 133.65 kg
8 lb = 3.63 kg	8 stone = 50.80 kg	22 stone = 139.70 kg
9 lb = 4.08 kg	9 stone = 57.15 kg	23 stone = 146.05 kg
10 lb = 4.54 kg	10 stone = 63.50 kg	24 stone = 152.40 kg
11 lb = 4.99 kg	11 stone = 69.85 kg	25 stone = 158.75 kg
12 lb = 5.44 kg	12 stone = 76.20 kg	26 stone = 165.10 kg
13 lb = 5.90 kg	13 stone = 82.55 kg	27 stone = 171.45 kg
14 lb = 6.35 kg	14 stone = 88.90 kg	28 stone = 177.80 kg

Ideal body weight and average height ratios for infants and children

Age	Ideal body weight		Average height	
	kg	lb	cm	in
Newborn (full term)	3.5	7.7	50	20
1 month	4.2	9	55	22
3 months	5.6	12	59	23
6 months	7.7	17	67	26
1 year	10	22	76	30
3 years	15	33	94	37
5 years	18	40	108	42
7 years	23	51	120	47
12 years	39	86	148	58
Adult				
Male	68	150	173	68
Female	56	123	163	64

Height

Imperial	Metric (cm)	Imperial	Metric (cm)
4'8"	142	5'6"	167.5
4'9"	144.5	5'7"	170
4'10"	147	5'8"	172.5
4'11"	150	5'9"	175
5'	152.5	5'10"	177.5
5'1"	155	5'11"	180
5'2"	157.5	6'	183
5'3"	160	6'1"	185.5
5'4"	162.5	6'2"	188
5'5"	165	6'3"	190.5

Child development chart

Age	Motor development	Social skills
2 months	Can lift head when prone	Recognizes a familiar face
3 months	Can hold head erect	Laughs out loud and smiles at
4 months	Can hold head still when sitting	mother
5 months	Can roll from back to tummy and vice versa	Reaches out to people
		Can discriminate between family
6 months	Can lift cup by handle and sit without support	and strangers
		Starting to imitate sounds
7 months	Able to stand with help	Can play peek a boo
8 months	Can feed self with fingers	Shows fear of strangers
9 months	Crawling and pulling self to standing position	Starting to imitate simple acts
		Is shy with strangers
10 months	Can pick up objects	Opens arms to be picked up
	Sits by falling	Cries when chastised
11 months	Pushes toys and tries to walk unaided	Waves bye bye
		Responds to own name when
12 months	Hand dominance becomes apparent	called
		Imitates vocal sounds
	Walks with help	Knows own name
	Uses spoon to feed self	Shakes head for 'No'
15 months	Can walk short distances unaided	Does things to attract attention
18 months	Can throw a ball	Tries to help when dressing
2 years	Can stack a tower of 6 cubes	Can point to objects
3 years	Dresses without supervision	Follows directions
	Can balance on one foot for a few seconds	Separates from mother easily
		Copies others
4 years	Can catch a bounced ball	Can recognize colours
5 years	Can draw a simple picture of a man	Can define some words
	Can walk backwards	Social skills continue to develop

Body mass index

Body mass index (BMI) is used to determine whether an individual, male or female, falls into a broad band considered to be of a healthy weight or is outside the parameters deemed to be healthy. It is also used by scientists and researchers to determine the health implications of being a certain BMI.

Classifications are as follows:

- underweight   BMI < 20
- normal weight   BMI 20-25
- overweight   BMI 25-30
- obese   BMI > 30

English formula

BMI = (weight in pounds ÷ height in inches ÷ height in inches) × 703

For example: A person weighing 210 pounds and standing 6 feet tall would have a BMI = 210 pounds divided by 72 inches divided by 72 inches multiplied by 703 = 28.5.

Metric formula

BMI = weight in kilograms ÷ (height in metres)^2

or

BMI = (weight in kilograms ÷ height in cms ÷ height in cms) × 10,000

For example: A person weighing 95.3 kilograms and standing 182.9 centimetres tall would have a BMI = 95.3 kg divided by 182.9 cm multiplied by 10,000 = 28.5.

Laboratory values

General clinical chemistry reference ranges

Sodium	130-147 mmol/L
Potassium	3.3-5.5 mmol/L
Bicarbonate	22-32 mmol/L
Chloride	95-107 mmol/L
Urea	1.7-8.3 mmol/L
Creatinine	53-106 µmol/L
Total protein	66-87 g/L
Albumin	38-51 g/L
(Globulin)	16-33 g/L
Calcium	2.02-2.60 mmol/L
(Adjusted calcium)	2.02-2.60 mmol/L
Phosphate	0.80-1.60 mmol/L
Alkaline phosphate	60-306 µ/L
Total bilirubin	0-19 µmol/L
AST	10-34 µ/L
ALT	7-33 µ/L
GGT	7-49 µ/L
LDH	120-450 µ/L
CPK	25-190 µ/L
Glucose (non-fasting)	3.0-11.0 mmol/L
Protein (total)	66-87 g/L
Magnesium	0.8-1.00 mmol/L
Uric acid	140-420 µmol/L
Amylase	0-90 µ/L

Lipid ranges

Triglycerides		0.5-2.2 mmol/L
HDL	Male	1.0-1.5 mmol/L
	Female	1.2-1.7 mmol/L
LDL	Male	1.7-5.4 mmol/L
	Female	1.5-5.8 mmol/L

Cholesterol WHO risk limits

Age	Moderate risk	High risk
20-29	> 5.2	> 5.6
30-39	> 5.7	> 6.2
over 40	> 6.2	> 6.7

Normal haematology values

Haemoglobin (Hb)	Adult: 13.5-18 g/dL	Child: 5/12-1 yr: 10-15 g/dL; 5-14 yrs: 11-16 g/dL
Packed-cell volume (PCV)	41%	
White cell count (WCC)	Adult: 4.0-10.0 x 10^9/L	Child: 2 yrs 6.0-17x 10^9/L
WCC differential:		
• Neutrophils	Adult: 60-70%	Child: 1 yr 32%; newborn 61%
• Lymphocytes	Adult: 23-35%	Child: 6 yrs 42%; 12 yrs 38%
• Monocytes	Adult: 4-8%	Child: 1-12 yrs 4-8%
• Eosinophils	1-4%	
• Basophils	0.4-1%	
Platelets	Adult and child: 150-400 x 10^9/L	
Leucocytes	4.0-11.0 x 10^9/L	
Red blood cell count (RBC)	4.6-6.0 x 10^{12} (million/μL)	
Mean corpuscular haemoglobin (MCH)	30-35 pg	
Mean corpuscular volume (MCV)	75-95 fl	
Mean corpuscular haemoglobin concentration (MCHC)	0.32-0.36 g/dL	

Coagulation tests

Prothrombin time	Adult: 11-15 secs
Fibrinogen	200-400 mg/dL
Bleeding time	1-3 mins

Arterial blood gases

Adult	Child
pH 7.35-7.45	pH 7.36-7.44
$PaCO_2$ 35-45 mmHg	All other measurements are the same as adult
PaO_2 75-100 mmHg	
HCO_3 24-28 mEq/L	

Calculating infusion (drip) rates

The rate of administration of a continuous or intermittent infusion may be calculated from the following equation:

$$\frac{\text{Number millilitres to be infused}}{\text{Number hours over which infusion is to be delivered}} \times \frac{\text{Number drops per millilitre}}{60 \text{ minutes}} = \text{Number drops to be delivered per minute}$$

In this equation, 60 is a factor for the conversion of the number of hours to the number of minutes; the number of drops per millilitre is dependent on the administration set used and the viscosity of the infusion fluid. The number of drops per minute can usually be found on the solution set packaging.

For example, crystalloid fluid administered via a solution set is delivered at the rate of 20 drops/ml whilst the rate of packed red cells given via a blood transfusion administration set should be calculated at 15 drops/ml.

- A solution set with crystalloids (e.g. normal saline) = 20 drops/ml
- A blood-giving set with blood or blood products = 15 drops/ml

Examples

Anne is to be given 500 ml of normal saline over four hours. The calculation would be:

$$\frac{500 \text{ ml}}{4} \times \frac{20}{60} = 41.66 \text{ (42) drops per minute}$$

John is to be given one unit of blood over three hours. The unit of blood has a volume of 300 ml. The calculation would be:

$$\frac{300 \text{ml}}{3} \times \frac{15}{60} = 25 \text{ drops per minute}$$

Calculating medications

Medicines are prescribed and dispensed in a variety of forms dependent on the drug itself, its degree of stability and its mode of action. Client preference is also considered if at all possible. Regardless of route they are normally measured by metric weight, that is, grams (gms), milligrams (mgs) or micrograms (mcgs) (see Example 1). Some medicines may need to be dispensed in a solution, in which case these are prescribed by concentration, for example milligrams per millilitre (see Example 2).

> **Example 1:**
> Prednisolone 5 mgs orally BD (or twice a day)
> Digoxin 62.5 mcgs orally OD (or once a day)
>
> **Example 2:**
> Pholcodine 5 mgs/5 mls orally TDS (three times a day)

Sometimes you may need to convert a quantity from one unit into another. It is therefore important to remember that:

> 1 gram = 1000 milligrams and 1 milligram = 1000 micrograms
> 1 gram therefore = 1,000,000 micrograms

Given the potential for over-dosage when dealing with so many noughts it is easy to see why being able to calculate dosages is an essential function of a registered practitioner. So, let's get calculating ...

Converting 250 mgs into grams

The mgs need to be changed to gm, that is, one thousand times bigger, so the number (250) must be made one thousand times smaller to compensate. The easiest way to do this is to decimalize it, i.e. 250.0, and then moving the decimal point three places to the left = 0.250, which is generally written 0.25.

> 250 mgs therefore equals 0.25 gms

To convert the opposite way, i.e. gms to mgs, you would reverse the process. For example 0.5 gms = 500 mgs.

When administering medication you will probably be given the *total* dose a client is to receive. You must then determine how much of the drug is in each tablet or preparation and then calculate how many tablets the client will need.

For example: Fred is prescribed 60 mgs of Prednisolone and the tablets available are 5 mgs each. How many tablets would you need to give Fred?

You need to determine how many 5 mgs are in 60 mgs. That means dividing 60 by 5, that is:

$$\frac{\text{The amount you want (60)}}{\text{The amount you've got (5)}}$$

Fred would therefore need 12 tablets. This seems a lot of tablets so if you are ever in doubt, even when qualified, always check with a colleague. It is always better to be safe rather than sorry.

But what if Fred is prescribed 1.5 gms of a drug which is only available in 500 mg tablets?

You first need to convert the gms to mgs, that is, 1.5 gms = 1500 mgs.

Then divide the amount you want by the amount you have, that is, $\frac{1500}{500}$. Fred therefore needs 3 tablets.

When administering liquids we can easily adapt our formula. For example, Fred needs 75 mgs and the drug comes as 25 mgs/5 mls

$$\frac{75 \text{ mgs}}{25 \text{ mgs in 5 mls}} = 3 \times 5 \text{ mls}$$

Fred therefore needs 15 mls.

If Fred needs an injection of 80 mgs, and the solution is 60 mgs/ml and the ampoule contains 5 mls:

$$\frac{80 \text{ mgs}}{50 \text{ mgs in 1 ml}} = 1.6 \text{ mls}$$

You would therefore need to draw up 1.6 mls and discard 3.4 mls.

Record of achievement

Penelope Ann Hilton

Guidelines on the use of this record of achievement

This record section is designed to help you direct your learning in relation to development of your clinical skills and assist you in keeping a record of your progress. You may find it is useful in providing additional evidence for your professional portfolio. It lists the core skills addressed within the main text. Clearly the list of skills is not exhaustive, and in recognition of this fact spaces are included for you to add any skills unique to your personal learning experiences.

It is suggested that you initial and date the first column when you have been instructed in or studied the theoretical underpinnings of the skill, and initial and date the other columns when:

Level 1 - You have observed the procedure in the practice setting

Level 2 - You have participated in the skill under direct supervision

Level 3 - You have performed the skill on a number of occasions and now require minimal supervision

Level 4 - You can perform the skill safely and competently, giving the rationale for your actions

Level 5 - You have taught the skill to others.

It is recommended that initials denoting achievement of Levels 4 and 5 be those of a registered nurse assessor, though this will clearly require local negotiation as this document is not intended to circumvent your locally determined summative assessment(s) of practice.

When performing each skill, remember that it is important to exhibit not only the psychomotor element but also the affective and cognitive components (i.e. attitude and knowledge).

Skills related to the activity of breathing

Skill	Instructed/Studied	1	2	3	4	5
Assess individual's ability to breathe normally						
Monitor and record respiratory rate						
Monitor and record peak flow						
Maintain airway of:						
infant						
child						
adult						
Monitor and record expectorant						
Safely dispose of sputum secretions						
Obtain sputum specimen						
Maintain safe administration of oxygen as prescribed via:						
mask						
nasal cannula						
humidifier						
Perform rescue breathing (artificial respiration):						
infant/child/adult						

Skills related to the activity of mobility

Skill	Instructed/Studied	1	2	3	4	5
Assess individual's ability to mobilize safely						
Care of self						
Assess task, individual capacity, load and environment						
Move inanimate objects						
Moving and handling of a range of clients into the following positions:						
upright						
recumbent						
semi-recumbent						
lateral						
semi-prone (recovery)						
prone						
side to side						
Move a range of clients from:						
chair to chair						
bed to chair						
chair to bed						
up the bed						
up in the chair						
cot						
Care for an individual who is falling						
Care for an individual who has fallen						

Skills related to the activity of personal cleansing and dressing

Skill	Instructed/Studied	1	2	3	4	5

Make a bed/cot that is:
    unoccupied
    occupied						

Changing a sheet on an occupied bed:
    top to bottom
    side to side						

Dispose of linen which is:
    uncontaminated
    contaminated						

Assist individuals requiring a:
    shower
    general bath
    wash
    bed bath						

Assist individuals maintain their
    oral hygiene:
        cleansing of teeth/dentures/
            mucous membranes
        use of mouthwashes/dental floss/
            interdental sticks						

Administration of eye care						

Facial shaving:
    with a safety razor
    with an electric shaver						

Care of hair:
    washing in bed
    dealing with infestation						

Assist a variety of individuals to
    dress:
        infant
        child
        adult						

Skills related to the activity of maintaining a safe environment

Skill	Instructed/Studied	1	2	3	4	5
Universal precautions - effective: handwashing use of gloves use of plastic aprons safe disposal of equipment						
Adheres to Health and Safety at Work Act in relation to: disinfection policies disposal of infected materials dealing with mercury spillage dealing with blood and body fluids radiation reporting untoward occurrences						
Perform a simple dressing using aseptic technique						
Obtain a wound swab						
Monitor pulse: radial carotid apex femoral						
Monitor and record blood pressure using: a mercury sphygmomanometer an aneroid sphygmomanometer an electronic device						
Administration of medicines (under direct supervision in keeping with trust policies):						
Ensures safe storage of medicines						
Respond in the event of an actual or suspected fire						
Respond in the event of a cardiac arrest						
Respond in the event of other emergency (state type):						

Skills related to the activity of eating and drinking

Skill	Instructed/Studied	1	2	3	4	5
Assess individual's nutritional status						
Assist clients in selecting appropriate meals/fluids						
Monitor and record nutritional intake						
Monitor and record fluid balance						
Assist clients with feeding						
Assist clients with drinking						
Feed dependent clients						
Recognize and report changes in client's condition						
Provide first aid to a client who is choking						

Skills related to the activity of communicating

Skill	Instructed/Studied	1	2	3	4	5
Respond appropriately to telephone calls						
Assess the communication needs of clients						
Communicate effectively with clients who have a: hearing difficulty speaking difficulty language difficulty comprehension difficulty						
Manage a client exhibiting an aggressive outburst						
Recognize and report changes in client's condition						
Give and receive reports of client's condition: verbal written						

Skills related to the activity of dying

Skill	Instructed/Studied	1	2	3	4	5
Communicate with dying clients						
Communicate with relatives of dying clients						
Communicate with the bereaved						
Perform Last Offices						

Skills related to the activity of eliminating

Skill	Instructed/Studied	1	2	3	4	5
Assess individual's ability to eliminate effectively						
Assist clients to use: bedpan urinal toilet/commode						
Apply/change a nappy						
Empty a catheter bag						
Monitor and record urinary output						
Monitor and record bowel actions						
Monitor and record vomit/gastric aspirate						
Obtain specimen of urine/faeces/ vomit for laboratory examination						
Identify and report changes in client's condition						

Skills related to the activity of maintaining body temperature

Skill	Instructed/Studied	1	2	3	4	5
Assess an individual's ability to maintain a normal body temperature						
Assist individuals to select suitable attire to maintain a normal body temperature						
Monitor and accurately record the temperature of a: 　infant 　child 　adult via the following routes: 　orally 　axillary 　aurally 　using fever strips						
Use appropriate strategies to raise body temperature						
Use appropriate strategies to lower body temperature						
Participate in the assessment of client's ability to maintain body temperature						

Skills related to the activity of expressing sexuality

Skill	Instructed/Studied	1	2	3	4	5
Maintain privacy and dignity						
Assess individual's ability to express their sexuality: 　child 　adult						
Assist individuals to express their sexuality: 　child 　adult						

Skills related to the activity of working and playing

Skill	Instructed/Studied	1	2	3	4	5
Assess individual's ability to work and play						
Assist individuals to select appropriate work activities						
Assist individuals to select appropriate recreational activities						

Skills related to the activity of sleep and rest

Skill	Instructed/Studied	1	2	3	4	5
Assess individual's needs related to sleep and rest						
Monitor and record individual's sleep and rest patterns						
Assist individuals to achieve a balance between activity and rest						

Additional skills

Skill	Instructed/Studied	1	2	3	4	5

Adapted from Hilton PA (1996) *Clinical Skills Map* and reproduced with the kind permission of the University of Sheffield.

Index